Julian Norton qualified as a veterinary surgeon from Cambridge Veterinary School in 1996. He has spent most of his working life in his beloved North Yorkshire, at Skeldale Veterinary Centre — the modern relocated Herriot practice featured in the *All Creatures Great and Small* books. In 2015, the practice was made the subject of a television programme, which is now in its third series.

Outside of work, Julian is a keen triathlete and ski mountaineer. He has represented Team GB at age-group level for both middle-distance triathlon and long-course duathlon. He is married to Anne, also a veterinary surgeon, and has two sons, Jack and Archie; a Jack Russell terrier called Emmy; two guinea pigs called Sparkle and Shine; and a rabbit called Luna.

He is usually busy.

A YORKSHIRE VET THROUGH THE SEASONS

Julian Norton has been a vet for over twenty years, and in that time he has treated animals of every kind — snakes and lizards, fish and fowl, sheep, goats, alpacas, cows, horses — you name it, Julian has seen it and, most likely, made it better. In *A Yorkshire Vet Through the Seasons*, Julian recounts more inspirational tales from his life, the animals he has treated and the people he has met, including the challenges and surprises that occur at the most unlikely times. Whether he is tending to a domestic pet at his practice in Thirsk, or called out to an injured swan in the middle of a cold Yorkshire night, the animals always come first, and Julian's passion and commitment are always to the fore.

Books by Julian Norton
Published by Ulverscroft:

HORSES, HEIFERS AND HAIRY PIGS

JULIAN NORTON

◆

A YORKSHIRE VET THROUGH THE SEASONS

Complete and Unabridged

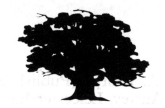

CHARNWOOD
Leicester

First published in Great Britain in 2017 by
Michael O'Mara Books Limited
London

First Charnwood Edition
published 2018
by arrangement with
Michael O'Mara Books Limited
London

A catalogue record for this book is available
from the British Library.

ISBN 978–1–4448–3744–5

For Anne, Jack and Archie

Contents

Introduction

The three adolescent alpacas looked very much happier and healthier as I pulled away from Jackie's farm. I had arrived an hour and a half earlier, after a panicked call from Jackie. The greedy youngsters had broken into the feed store and gorged themselves. All three were suffering from a severe condition called 'choke', in which the dry food swells as it absorbs moisture and gets stuck in the oesophagus.

After much anxiety and the passing of a stomach tube and lots of water to flush out the offending obstruction in each animal, I headed back towards Thirsk, to enjoy what was left of the brief time that is called 'lunch'. It was a lovely, mild autumn day and the sun was shining. My faithful Jack Russell terrier, Emmy, wagged her tail excitedly as we meandered down the familiar winding roads. At the end of a long track, I pulled over. I could not resist a short walk with my dog. It would also give me an opportunity to make the long overdue phone call to David, my book agent. He had been leaving messages for a week or so. My first book, *Horses, Heifers and Hairy Pigs: The Life of a Yorkshire Vet*, was proving popular, so I thought I knew what he was going to say when we eventually managed to have a conversation.

When my mobile phone finally connected, he launched straight in.

1

'Julian, we really think it would be a great idea if you could do another book.'

'Well, David, that's very easy for you to say,' I objected, as I found a tree stump to sit on. Emmy scurried in and out of the bushes, looking for adventures. 'It's not you who has to find the words . . . and the time!'

It wasn't that I didn't think I *could* write a second book, it was just that I wasn't sure I would have enough to say. I briefly laid out what I thought might work — a collection of veterinary anecdotes loosely based around the changing seasons, rather than the chronological memoir of my first book. David loved the idea and, before I had left my tree stump, I had apparently agreed to embark on the project that became known as *A Yorkshire Vet Through the Seasons*. I paused for a few moments to enjoy the tranquil scene that was the view towards Husthwaite, a pretty little village nearby. I had just committed myself and my family to another six months or more of late nights, early mornings, edits, rethinks and chapters in the bin. But I knew it would be worthwhile.

This book, like the first, has been a combined effort, with much hard work from my wife, Anne, who skilfully edited every word. She rearranged, rewrote and reread until she was sure it was a good read. My oldest son, Jack, who also has a keen eye for detail, is responsible for the brilliant photograph on the front cover. He asked me one Sunday evening, as he was finishing his school work and I was scratching my head over another section, 'Dad, do you like writing books?' He must have noticed my furrowed brow and expected a negative answer, but I replied that writing a book is exactly like doing homework. Sometimes it is great. Sometimes it is a pain in the neck. But, when it's finished and you are satisfied with your achievement, then it's blooming brilliant. I hope this comes across in this book and I hope that it will bring as much enjoyment to you, the reader, as it has to me, as I have rekindled my stories and thought back over all the amazing people and their amazing animals that I have encountered and treated during my life as a veterinary surgeon in rural North Yorkshire.

WINTER

The warmth had yet to return to my fingers and toes as my car slid, slowly and gently but completely out of control, down to the bottom of the hill, towards the village of Boltby. It was deepest winter and my day had started with an early-morning call to calve a heifer at a wild and remote farm, way up in the middle of the moors. There had been a lot of snow and it was bitterly cold. Most of the roads had been cleared but the icy patches at the bottom of this hill took me by surprise. The drifts of snow piled up on each side of the road afforded some protection and I slithered to a pillowy halt in a snow-laden hedge. The car was unscathed and so was I. I needed to avoid any further accidents like this if I was to get to my next call — a cow that was down with milk fever — in Pickhill on the far side of the river Swale. Cautiously, I made my way along the winding lanes, down from the wintery hills and into the icy fog of the Vale of York. I'd rushed out of the house without even a cup of tea, and my warm bed seemed a world away. For a vet in rural North Yorkshire, winter could be a tough time of year . . .

Swanny

'Okay. So it actually came to your door, and knocked on it?'

It was the end of November and evening surgery was unusually quiet. Our receptionist, Sylvia, was on the phone. She has an amazing knack of painting a picture using one half of a telephone conversation, allowing the vet, hovering within earshot, to get an idea of what might be required. Listening to Sylvia's commentary this evening, I could tell that it was something out of the ordinary.

'Okay . . . And it's lifting its leg off the ground? . . .

'Right . . . And where is it now? . . .

'Oh! It's gone back to the lake?'

Even with this excellent narrative, I was struggling to work out what the evening might have in store for me.

The lady on the phone lived next to a fishing lake on the outskirts of town. There are a number of small lakes like this around Thirsk. They were once clay pits, dug to collect clay to make bricks. The brick kilns are long gone now, and the abandoned pits have filled up with water. Enterprising landowners have realized that stocking them with fish provides an excellent way to attract fishermen, who come from miles around. If you own a fishing lake it offers a much more lucrative way to pay the bills than farming cattle.

The lady explained to Sylvia that the family tea had been interrupted by a knock on the door. To her astonishment, the visitors were two black swans standing side by side on the doorstep. One was a male, slighter larger, and the other was a small female. The female swan was holding her left leg off the ground and was clearly distressed. It appeared they had come up to the house to ask for help. However, as the phone call progressed, both birds had disappeared back into the darkness, to the relative safety of the lake.

How on earth was I going to find an injured black swan on a dark lake?

And even if I could find it, how was I going to catch it?

With some trepidation I collected up the various pieces of equipment I thought I might need. I had never captured a swan before, and the tales of their wings being powerful enough to break a man's arm did nothing to help my confidence. I canvassed opinion from other members of staff, but no one could come up with any helpful suggestions. There were various comments about how delicate their necks were, and that the use of a net was out of the question, because of the risk of damage to the feathers.

I definitely needed an assistant. Luckily, Sarah, our proficient and dynamic head nurse, was quick to volunteer. This was partly because she relished a challenge, but also because it was an escape from the tedious job of counting out tablets during evening surgery. So, armed with a range of equipment — a net (we decided to take it just in case despite the risk of feather damage), some large blankets, a dogcatcher contraption (usually employed for grabbing dangerous dogs) and even a duvet cover — we piled into the practice van and set off.

Even though it was only just after five in the evening, it was already very dark. Darkness descends quickly in Thirsk at the onset of winter. We live in the very north of North Yorkshire, only twenty miles from the county's northernmost town of Yarm, where the River Tees forms Yorkshire's border with County Durham. Hailing, as I do, from West Yorkshire, I always used to think that places like Harrogate, Ilkley, Ripon and Skipton were 'northern' Yorkshire towns, but Thirsk is some way beyond those places. As a result, we enjoy lovely long summer evenings, but at the opposite end of the year, as it was tonight, the winter nights start at four o'clock in the afternoon.

As we trundled out of the practice in the darkness, I couldn't help thinking that the next hour or so would be a complete waste of time. The two swans would be swimming in the middle of a pitch-black lake, out of sight and certainly out of the grasp of a veterinary surgeon and his nurse, even if they were armed with a long pole in the form of a dogcatcher. I had wellies, but they were only standard length, so I would not be able to wade very far from the edge without getting wet feet. I had visions of the swans simply gliding away into the night.

There was a long and even darker lane that led us to a car park, where we met the lady who had made the emergency call. Her daughter (as every good child with a mobile phone does these days) had filmed the swans as they knocked on the glass door. She showed me her phone and sure enough, there they were — two swans standing on the doorstep, the female looking anxious, while the male pecked with its beak on the door to attract attention. This touching image made Sarah and me determined to capture the injured bird. If we could grab the patient and transfer her safely to the back of the van, we could take her back to the practice and attempt to treat her injured leg.

So, armed with the various paraphernalia we thought might be helpful, we made our way by torchlight to the lake. After about five minutes of fumbling around in the dark, we found the water's edge, just in time to see the two birds sliding into the black depths.

'Bother', was my first thought. Once the birds had taken to the water, we knew they had the edge over us. As I was trying to hatch a plan, Sarah realized that the birds would soon be out of sight. Without any discussion or warning, or concern about the depth of the water, she launched herself at the nearest swan and grabbed it, throwing her arms around its body and wings. We had discussed our tactics on the way to the lake, but this wasn't what we had in mind. Sarah's instincts had got the better of her, but luckily for everyone, including the swan, it paid off. I helped her out of the water, a swan in her arms and a massive grin on her face. Good fortune was in our favour, as the swan that Sarah had grabbed was, indeed, the one with the injured leg. Stage one of our evening's adventure was complete and she had done a brilliant job.

It didn't take long to establish the cause of the problem. In the light of my torch, I could see that this elegant bird had a fishing hook embedded in her left leg. It was very deep and very well attached, and there was no way I could remove it without a general anaesthetic and surgical equipment.

By now the swan was starting to feel a bit fed up with our rescue attempt and was flapping and making a great commotion. She didn't realize that we were trying to help. All she wanted was to escape, and return to her partner in the water. For his part, he had decided that this was a horrific nocturnal kidnapping attempt and he was trying to chase us away. It was impossible to explain to the birds that we were here to help and that all would be well, once we had done our work. So it took some struggling and the help of a large blanket to bundle her safely into the van. We sometimes like to call it the 'Animal Ambulance', but it is, in fact, just a van.

By the time we got back to the practice, she was a very cross swan. Not only was she in great pain, but she had been kidnapped and then shaken around in the back of the van for quarter of an hour. There was every reason to be cross. Sarah was, however, soon in control of the situation, and we transferred the bird to the operating theatre where we wasted no time in getting her asleep under anaesthetic. Usually, by this point with wildlife or stray animals, we have given the patient a name. It makes life easier, not least because we can then write a name on its hospital record sheets and on the kennel where it recovers after its operation. In this case, all we could think of was 'Swanny'. It seemed apt enough and soon Swanny was fast asleep on the operating table as the gas took its effect.

At last I could have a proper look at the damage. There was a large hook embedded deeply in her leg. It had penetrated right down to the bone and, as I investigated with my scalpel, I discovered that it was also wrapped tightly around the main artery going down the leg to the foot. Water birds have big blood vessels in their legs, and the artery and vein run very closely together. This is a special adaptation for conserving core body heat, called the 'counter current heat exchange'. Heat from the warm arterial blood coming from the body warms up the cool blood in the veins. This means that the feet do not get too cold when the swan (or duck, or goose or moorhen) is swimming around in very cold water, but also, crucially, that the body temperature does not drop too low as a result of cold blood returning to the core. You or I would get icy feet if we spent our winters paddling around in a lake, and very quickly develop hypothermia, but because of this special arrangement of artery and vein, water birds can cope very well. However, right now it made my job more difficult. I had two big and important blood vessels to preserve to avoid major haemorrhage and to ensure Swanny would have a nice warm left foot for the rest of her winter!

The only way to remove the hook safely and without causing further injury was to cut it in half. Fishhooks are sometimes barbed, which means they cannot be pulled out the way they went in. Pulling on them simply embeds them more deeply in the tissue and can cause terrible tissue damage. Using cutters usually employed for trimming the metal pins during fracture repair, I managed to snip the hook just in front of the barb. Once that was done, the barbed part lifted away, and I could gently pull the remainder of the hook out, with minimal further trauma. Thankfully, those important blood vessels remained intact. I stitched the wound with dissolving suture material — there was not a chance we would be seeing Swanny at the surgery again to take the stitches out, as we would with our usual patients.

After administering painkilling injections and antibiotics to treat infection, Swanny was put into her kennel for the evening. This was easier said than done because a semi-anaesthetized swan has no control over its very long neck. Swanny's head was floppy and out of control. Sarah and I had to be very careful not to let it fall into the wrong position. The last thing she wanted was to wake up with a sore neck! The plan was to release Swanny back to her mate in the lake the following morning, but first she needed to recover from the operation, so she settled down for a peaceful but lonely night.

The next day was a Friday. Fridays are always very busy at the practice, so Sarah suggested we should come in early to make the journey to the lake before the bustle of the day started. We knew it would be a two-person job again and that it would take some time to manhandle Swanny back into the van. We arranged to meet at the practice at seven o'clock.

Swanny had enjoyed a quiet but rather unusual night in a dog kennel, resting on a thick duvet rather than her usual nest of reeds. Unsurprisingly, she was somewhat annoyed by the time we arrived in the morning. Sarah (who was now accomplished at grabbing swans) grappled her out of the kennel and I applied a liberal coating of Vaseline to the wound, to protect it from the muddy water. It would only last for a short time, but I reasoned any extra assistance to stop infection would be helpful. We were soon back in the van and heading to the lake.

The weak, winter sun was just beginning to emerge as we took Swanny back towards the spot where we had captured her the previous evening. It looked very different in daylight and it became evident that Sarah had been extremely lucky to plunge in where she did. A few metres to either side the water was much deeper, and she would have been up to her neck!

We peered through the mist, across the water, for any sign of the male swan. Nothing to be seen. There were a few noises from other water birds as they made their first morning calls, but no swan. Had Swanny's mate left the lake to look for his lifelong companion? This would be dreadfully unlucky, we thought, but he did look very upset when he had seen Swanny being

14

ambushed and bundled into a van which sped off into the night. Who could blame him for going to search for her? The people who lived in the house near the lake, who had called us in the first place, came out to meet us and reassured us that they would send out a search party if necessary. Right now, though, we had to release our patient. She, at least, was desperate to get back to the water.

Swans are very graceful when they are on the water, but not graceful at all when they are walking on land. Swanny lumbered along to the lake in a very ungainly fashion, then fell headlong into the water with an undignified splash. After this initial dunking though, she did look pleased. We all held our breath, as she regained her confidence and took a few tentative dips of her head into the water, as if to wash away the veterinary smells that she had picked up from the surgery. As the sun rose over the lake, it was a wonderful sight. The bird was clearly delighted to be back where she belonged.

Then, from the far side of the lake, the male swan appeared. He made his way very slowly, but very purposefully, to near where we were standing and directly towards Swanny. As the two birds got close together, the male let out a peculiar noise, as if to say, 'Thank goodness you're back. I didn't know where you had gone.' Then the most amazing thing happened. The two swans entwined their necks, and, silhouetted against the rising sun, this embrace made a perfect heart shape.

Swanny had made a fantastic recovery and it

was wonderful to see her back where she belonged and happy with her mate. This type of work is very rewarding, and there is an unwritten agreement amongst veterinary surgeons that we will all do whatever we can for injured wildlife, absorbing the costs ourselves. So, much as it was lovely watching the two swans swim off together, my morning appointment list was beckoning and I could put it off no longer.

The swans glided into the distance, away from us and into the sun. For the onlookers on the bank, it was the perfect way to start the day.

16

Malcolm

November was always the month for my annual inspection of Malcolm's racing greyhound kennel. Malcolm was a larger-than-life character, and I came to know him well over the years. Not only was he a successful greyhound owner and trainer, but he was also the proprietor of a roadside café near Thirsk. It is difficult to describe the man properly. He had the appearance and sense of humour of the 1980s comedian Les Dawson, and was a kind man and a loyal friend. He was bursting with energy. Behind the grill of his café, he could flip a fried egg with abandon whilst holding an animated conversation on the mobile phone that was perennially glued to his right ear. However, it was the passion he held for his dogs that stood out more than anything to me, and it was through his greyhounds that I knew him.

Aside from his annual inspection, there were regular visits to check the dogs, to confirm that they were in the best of health and in peak condition. Behind the counter of the café, amongst the plastic trays of mushrooms which were a vital ingredient in the enormous fried breakfasts Malcolm conjured up for hungry lorry drivers, were numerous trophies and photographs of handsome, winning dogs. For all his own lack of athleticism (although he had, apparently, been a semi-professional football

17

player for a team in South Yorkshire in his younger days), Malcolm obviously knew how to get his greyhounds to perform at the highest level. He was always looking to us, his vets, to confirm his latest idea, endorse his most novel feeding regime or comment upon the new potion that had been recommended by the Irish vet he had met at a race meeting.

The November inspection was always a cold affair, once the steaming environment of the café was left behind. On one occasion I left the café and walked into the most vigorous of storms. I was sure that the lorries parked in the enormous and distinctly uneven car park would soon be lying on their sides. Not a single leaf was left clinging to the trees, but all the kennels were warm and immaculate. I had to inspect each one, as well as checking on the health of the animals. Every kennel was deeply bedded in thick-piled carpet and paper shavings. The dogs were warmer than the humans, as each one had its own heat lamp, glowing red in the early winter gloom.

As I looked through the medicine book, to make sure all the greyhounds had been vaccinated at the right time and had received de-worming and flea treatment, Malcolm would keep up a running commentary, showing me his latest machine to massage the muscles of his dogs, presenting his newest treadmill or asking for my thoughts on his most recent tonic.

'Rocky! Look at this! It's from my mate in Ireland. His dog — beautiful dog he was, half brother to my old bitch — just came second in the Irish Derby. What d'ya reckon? It's supposed to improve the blood! Is it worth a go? What d'ya reckon? Any good or complete waste of time? I'll try it if you think it'll work.'

But before I could come up with an answer, Malcolm had always moved on to his next idea, usually a pot of tablets or a new vitamin supplement.

Malcolm always called me Rocky. He also called his dogs 'Rocky' or 'Rebel' or 'Flash'. These were their pet names, because the best dogs — those that made it past the 'flapping' tracks of the north of England — all had racing names. The only other pet names he would use for his dogs were 'Peter' or 'Julian'. Peter is my work colleague and the senior partner at our practice, Skeldale Veterinary Centre, in Thirsk. Peter and I were the only vets to whom Malcolm entrusted the care of his greyhounds, but he saved our names especially for those dogs which he perceived had no chance of winning anything. I could not imagine seeing a photo behind the counter at the café, emblazoned with the winner's name 'Peter' or 'Julian', although at this place, anything was possible!

There was greyhound miscellany in every direction and I was never surprised by any of the unusual things that I came across around the kennels. On one occasion I arrived to vaccinate a litter of puppies, all of which were, according to Malcolm, destined to be winners of the Derby when they grew older. Malcolm was sitting outside the kennels on a massive chair that was painted gold. It looked just like a throne. All he needed to complete the image was a crown, orb and sceptre. Instead he held a cigarette and a mug of tea. And, of course, his mobile phone.

On this inspection day though, there was no throne. After my usual perfunctory trawl through the checklist, peering into cabinets and scrutinizing records, we got onto the best bit — looking at the dogs. As always, the animals were handsome and healthy. Any instances of illness or injury were brought into the clinic immediately, with great urgency, always preceded by a loud telephone call from Malcolm, succinctly explaining the details of the problem. He expected Peter or me to see every ailment, however minor, within half an hour, which was the time it took him to lift the dog into the back of his estate car and race to the practice.

'Raight. I'll be there at half ten,' were his usual parting words, after which the line would go dead. All other work would have to be shuffled around to make way for the larger-than-life Malcolm and his poorly dog.

Happily, today nobody was ill. The dogs were paraded out one by one for me to inspect.

'Andre, fetch that brindle bitch from up top!' Malcolm would bellow at the Eastern European kennel lad, who looked about ninety years old and always wore a confused expression. Andre would saunter away and, belying his confused expression, would usually return with the correct animal.

Finally, the last dog was summoned.

'Rocky, can you bring me James?' Today's Rocky was Malcolm's son, who also helped out in the café and the kennels and was proudly following in his father's large footsteps. He wasn't called Rocky either — I think his name was Greg.

A beautiful adolescent black dog stood in front of me.

'That', pronounced Malcolm, 'is James.' He stood back with his hands on his hips, bursting with pride. 'James Pool.'

'Wow!' seemed the right response. He did indeed look handsome, but no more so than the other twenty-nine dogs I had just seen.

'That is a lovely dog — and an interesting name,' I commented.

'Well, Rocky' — Rocky being me, this time — 'we expect great things of him. His father won at Sheffield the other weekend. That's why we called him James Pool.'

'Okay. Who is James Pool?'

I had never heard of him.

'I don't know, but I thought it sounded like a grand name. The name of a winner!'

I admired and then inspected 'James Pool' with the thoroughness that Malcolm expected. He did seem splendid and, once he had eaten the right food and moved through the ranks, I assured Malcolm that I thought he was a future champion.

'Hey, Rocky. Look at this!'

'What now?' I thought. Was this to be an even more imperial greyhound, and if so, what on earth would this one be called? But I was not presented with another dog. Instead, I was ushered into the food preparation area. It was part of the kennel inspection process — I had to make sure the kitchen was clean and tidy, and that all the food was either in a fridge or a rat-proof container. However, Malcolm was not showing me his hygiene status. He was gesturing at a veritable mountain of meat, which was hiding under a tarpaulin on one of his kitchen units.

'That, Rocky, is pure, prime beef! That's got to be good for 'em, eh? Pure meat. No waste. What d'ya reckon? It's good stuff, you know!'

Its provenance was obscure, apart from that Malcolm knew a man who 'fetched it in a lorry all the way from Middlesbrough.' I tried to explain that the basis of a balanced diet for any dog, but especially a performance one, involved an intricate balance of calcium and phosphate that might not be met by this pure meat. But my cautionary words fell on deaf ears. Malcolm was back on his phone, no doubt organizing his next delivery of beef.

★ ★ ★

There is a common misconception that people who own a lot of animals must have a reduced affection for each individual. Surely it is impossible to have equal measures of affection for each of twenty dogs? For Malcolm, though, this could not have been further from the truth. Despite having many dogs at this time and many more previously, he treated each as his one and only beloved pet.

I saw him one morning after answering a

typical phone call from him, urging me to see his dog immediately. He had been racing at Sunderland the previous evening. The dog had pulled up on the final bend, finishing lame and last. The veterinary surgeon attending the track had patched up the hobbling greyhound with a bandage of monstrous proportions, which gave no indication of the extent of the injury underneath. I suspected it would be serious. So did Malcolm, although he always feared the worst.

I admitted the dog (this one called Flash) to our hospital, and set about rearranging my morning visits. Once this was done, I sedated him so that I could take off the huge bandage and examine his leg.

As I suspected, there was a large amount of swelling in his right hock, and instead of being held together firmly, there was a marked slackness to the joint. Before Malcolm and Flash had even appeared, I knew it would be the right hock that was the problem — it always is in a racing greyhound. The dogs run around the track in an anticlockwise direction, so the right hind is subject to most of the stress. It is the hock (the equivalent of our ankle joint) that bears the brunt of this stress. The joint comprises many small bones, held together very tightly and very specifically by ligaments, which keep everything in the right place. Even a tiny misalignment causes the joint to be painfully unstable and renders the dog very lame and unable to race. I took an x-ray, and it quickly became clear that one of the bones — the central tarsal bone — was severely out of position. It was either the end of Flash's racing days, or possibly even the end of his days altogether — most dog trainers do not even consider keeping a lame greyhound for a pet.

I telephoned Malcolm who answered immediately. I told him the bad news about the extent of the injury and the likely prognosis. Even if we operated, it was far from certain that the injury would heal well, and it would be complicated surgery. For most racing dogs, the outcome of this injury would not be a happy one, but Flash belonged to Malcolm.

'Well, he's been a good dog for me and he's a good mate. Do what you can for him. If he doesn't race again, I'll keep him as a pet. I'll pick him up this evening.' With that, characteristically, the phone went dead and I did not have the chance to explain the various potential complications and problems.

It was a good thing I had rearranged my morning's work because the repair of Flash's injury was both fiddly and time-consuming. I needed to cut over the joint, realign the bones that had been squeezed out of place and then, whilst keeping them in perfect alignment, apply a tiny bone screw to attach two of the bones to one another. This would keep them in place and stop the main central bone from slipping out of position.

The operation went well and Malcolm arrived that evening as promised, to collect his dog. Flash was bundled into the estate car, soon to be back to the luxury kennel and heat lamp from where he came.

A neat post-op x-ray, a tidy bandage, a happy dog and a firm handshake from Malcolm were all I needed to make this day another satisfying one.

'Thanks, Rocky! See ya next week!'

And with that he was off, mobile phone clamped back to his ear.

Out in all Weathers

The work of a veterinary surgeon in a mixed practice such as Skeldale is inextricably linked to the seasons. In some professions, people can be oblivious to the weather. The short walk to the car in the morning, the walk from the railway station to work, or the trip to the sandwich shop for lunch might be the only exposure they get to whatever is happening outside the office window.

In Thirsk, winter has set in by the end of November. The bitter cold is never far away, either in the dense fog that rolls up the Vale of York, or with the biting wind from the top of Sutton Bank. All the cattle are brought inside, not only to protect them from the harsh weather, but also to protect the fields, which would otherwise be churned up into muddy swamps. The grass is needed when spring comes back around and it is once again 'turnout' time.

But in November, with the cows all housed in farm sheds and buildings, and therefore much easier to handle, it is time to set about the list of jobs that has been saved up for this time. Dehorning of young stock, castration of calves, vaccination against pneumonia, trimming of hooves, blood testing and more are all to be done once the cows are in so, in this first part of the winter, the practice is very busy.

Whatever might be coming out of the sky, and from wherever the wind might be blowing, routine visits that have been arranged weeks in advance, often necessitating the drafting in of extra help, proceed whatever the weather. Through some sort of machismo on the part of the farmer or the vet, or both, we plough on regardless. No one wants to be accused of being soft.

The only time I can ever remember a job being cancelled on account of the weather was when the collecting yard at the farm was covered in a thick layer of ice, across which the cows would have found it impossible to walk without injury.

This was the winter during which arctic conditions descended over the whole country, from December 2009 until February the following year. It was also the winter during which John, who owned a beef suckler herd near Thirsk, had used a bull to serve all his cows that turned out to produce calves of enormous proportions. Every single calving was a challeng-ing job, and nearly all of them required assistance from the vet. The snow ploughs and gritters had abandoned the road to the farm in favour of the more frequented routes, so the four-mile journey down an icy Newsham Road was as much of a challenge as delivering the oversized calf at the other end.

The entries in John's wife's diary told the tale:

Saturday 26 December
Dogs out. Cattle checked. Geese fed.
Fire still burning in sitting room.
Silage to sheep in wood.

Bottled calf born last night (vet out).
Cow calved in New Shed overnight.
David and vet out at midday to cow calving.
Sandwiches for lunch.
Another cow calved in New Shed in after-
noon.
Did all outside jobs, cattle checked 11.30.
John up in night to check — 2 cows calved
in New Shed. Vet out again.

Sunday 27 December
Up at 4.45. Caesarian on cow in fold yard.
Live calf. Kicking cow.
Busy morning.
Vet and David here again by 10 a.m.
Children built snowman. Trixie frightened
of it!
Did feeding on my own — John snoozing
on sofa.
Two vets here. Two cows calving — both
caesarians.
Bottled new calf.
Bed at 12.30.
Fire in sitting room all day.

We were seeing an awful lot of John and his son David. Despite the terrible snowy conditions, the biggest challenge we faced was the unruly behaviour of the cows and heifers that needed our help. It is interesting that the diary entry only seemed to note that one of their cows was a 'kicking cow' because my recollection of this winter on Newsham Road was that nearly *all* the cows could be described in that way!

★ ★ ★

By mid December, it was always time for the annual pregnancy test on Alex's herd of Simmental cows. Everything about it was wild. The farm was in a wild place, up on the moors near Black Hambleton — a formidable hill on the Cleveland Way, where nothing much lives except grouse. Even the cows were wild, for they had spent their whole summer roaming on the edge of the moor.

All two hundred cows had just been rounded up and brought inside for winter. They had not been handled since they had produced their calves in the springtime. They were, therefore, quite cross. Their tempers were made worse by the fact that their calves, with which they had spent the last nine months, had been taken away that morning before sunrise. There was much mooing and bellowing and there were many attempts to escape. These big, strong cows were determined to get back to their calves and back out onto the moor. They were certainly not in the mood for veterinary attention.

It was always a tough day's work, starting early and finishing pretty much when the light disappeared. We would work constantly without a break even for coffee, let alone lunch. To stop would mean we would not be finished before dark, so I would always start the day of Alex's herd's pregnancy testing with a big breakfast and an extra pair of socks to keep out the cold.

The farm is lovely and traditional. The buildings are all made of solid blocks of Yorkshire

29

stone cut out of the nearby hills. There are extensive views to the moors beyond — when there is chance to see them, that is. There were no views to be had today. The angry cows were corralled in batches of about forty or fifty into a fold yard and then ushered down a corridor into a 'race' which was the width of just one cow, so that the animals couldn't turn around. The race led to a sliding wooden door, which in turn led to a metal cattle crush, where I did my thing — outside. It was conveniently positioned in the coldest part of the farm, in one of the draughtiest parts of North Yorkshire. The cold was made worse by the wind, which was blowing straight in from the north. The crush itself was freezing too, having been outside all night in sub-zero temperatures. There was no chance of the icy metal warming up in the sunshine either, since dark grey clouds hung menacingly around us.

As well as pregnancy testing each cow, which was the reason for my visit, I was also in charge of operating the crush to capture each one and keep her still, so she was safe to handle. There was a rhythm to the process — front door closed, bar in behind to stop the cow backing out, back door closed and locked, neck yoke closed, back door opened, bar removed, arm inserted into the cow's rectum to check for a calf. The whole process was then repeated in reverse after Alex had checked the ear tags. Each cow needed two and any missing ones, lost on the moorland over the summer, were replaced. The cow's bushy tail was clipped of extra hair, she was given her dose

30

of wormer and then released. Onto the next . . .

The important part of my job — the pregnancy testing — was lovely and warm. My arm was inserted into a temperature of exactly 101.5°F, which is the body temperature of a healthy cow, and it was much warmer than the outside temperature! So for thirty seconds or so of every five minutes, I would have a toasty warm right arm from fingers to shoulder. For the rest of the time my hands were in contact with either the cold air or the freezing metal of the cattle crush, which sapped all the warmth from my body.

But it was possibly my feet that were the coldest. I was moving around, but not much, and the concrete of the yard was icy. While the other tasks were being done with each cow, I was mainly standing still and the thin soles of my Wellington boots offered little barrier to the rising chill. That second pair of socks was a necessity.

By midday, however, we were progressing quite well and all serious problems had, so far, been avoided. Our assessment of how the day was going was judged not just by the percentage of cows pregnant, but also by the number of escapees and breakouts, and the number and extent of injuries to the assembled staff (kicks to the vet being the main one). Today, all was good.

Pregnancy testing provides crucial information for a farmer. The cows have been outside all summer, eating grass and allowing their spring-born calves to suckle and grow big and strong. A bull or two, or more, is introduced in mid-summer so the cows become pregnant ready to have another calf the following spring. Farming like this is not economically viable if each cow doesn't get close to producing one calf per year. Summer grazing is cheap if the farmer owns the land, but not if they have to rent the field. Winter food, grass silage, minerals and creep feed for the calves are all substantial costs that need to be covered, and for a beef suckler farmer like Alex, the sale of his calves is his only source of income.

If the cow is not pregnant, it is critical to find this out before winter. It is folly to feed an 'empty' cow all through the long winter months if she is not going to produce a baby in the spring. So, aside from this being a long, hard day for me, it is always a very important day for Alex and it can be stressful. Each time I shake my head to indicate the cow is 'empty', there is a noticeable drop in the mood. Conversely, when I cheerfully confirm that a cow is 'in calf', as I feel a foetus bobbing around inside the cow's uterus, the mood always lifts. I remember one day, when I was a student, following a veterinary surgeon who was pregnancy testing a group of about thirty cows. Not a single one was pregnant, and the farmer was just about in tears by the time we left the farm. It is not the fault of the vet, but as the harbingers of bad news, we always feel rather guilty at having to shake our head again. I dared not imagine what it would be like if that was the outcome today.

Happily, so far at least, that was not turning out to be the case. The problem that was becoming evident, however, as the day progressed, was the fragility of the wooden sliding door that was stopping cows coming out of the race, before being captured in the crush. The repeated opening and closing, which had to be done rapidly to stop the next animal bursting out, had taken its toll on the wood, which was already weak from its exposure to the elements. The door was becoming a shadow of its former self. Large splintered holes were appearing, one large enough for an impatient cow to stick its nose through.

Standing behind a cow with my arm inside its rectum, whilst warm, was not the safest place to be. A sudden twist to the left or right, or worse still downwards, could easily result in a debilitating injury to my elbow or shoulder. The deft accuracy of a kick from a cow's back legs does not need much further explanation, but now the integrity of the wooden door was the only thing stopping the next cow from bursting out and squashing me between it and the cow already in the crush. With my arm where it was, I had no way to escape. Should the wooden door fail under the weight and impatience of a 700-kilogram Simmental cow, I would be another statistic for the air ambulance and its team.

As the afternoon wore on, the frailty of the door was increasingly preying on my mind. The number of cows in the shed was slowly diminishing and the end of the day was becoming a real prospect, rather than a dim and distant pipe dream but, as the nose-sized hole grew into a hole big enough for a cow's head, my grounds for optimism receded.

It was at this point that the sleet started to come down. It had been threatening all day — dark, low cloud and a damp coldness that had risen from my feet as far as my knees and had stubbornly refused to dissipate during the afternoon. When you are working outside, sleet is the worst thing that can fall from the sky. Rain can be warm and snow, although colder in absolute temperature, does not penetrate so deeply. Sleet, however, is both freezing and somehow gets right through to your skin. It was slow at first, but it came down harder and harder, until the yard where we were working became covered in a silvery slush. It didn't stay silvery for long, as muck from the cows soon gave it a bronze sheen. The ground looked like a very unpalatable Slush Puppie drink.

Mercifully for everyone, the number of cows on the 'to do' side of the crush eventually dropped to single figures. Whilst this usually buoys the spirit, any experienced farmer or veterinary surgeon knows that this is not the time to start thinking of warm cups of tea. The last few cows are last for a very good reason — these are the ones who are best at evading capture. The cows left to test had avoided coercion into the race for the last six hours and they had no intention of going in now without a fight. Often the last ten cows can take as long to deal with as the first thirty, as they have much more space to run around in frustrating circles, and to pick up speed. At least chasing these last

34

few was out of the sleet and it was a good way of getting warm.

Two cows leapt over the gate to freedom. It is quite something to see a fully grown cow clear a four-foot gate from a standing start.

'Oh, bugger it, let's leave it at that,' were Alex's final words. We didn't know if they were pregnant, but he didn't look too bothered. It had been a tough day, and somehow, two escapees out of two hundred didn't seem too bad. And the door had held out.

Whilst I washed my wellies from the icy water butt near to where I had parked my car, we went through the numbers — 92 per cent were pregnant, not including the two escapees. This was not a bad result. Secretly, however, everyone was just relieved that the job was finished. We were all unscathed and still smiling. Just.

Smelly Cat

New Year's Eve is always the shortest straw to draw on the Christmas rota. Not only is it the one night of the year when everyone wants to socialize, but it is also the night we receive the most bizarre and unusual calls. This might be because clients, or animals — or both — have enjoyed the festivities just that little bit too much. It might, of course, just be coincidence.

One New Year's Eve call has gone down in history at the practice. It happened in the days before we were computerized, when patient records were kept on cards the size of a postcard. The card that recorded the clinical notes for this particular case has been kept for posterity. Without actually seeing it written in black and white, the story is almost impossible to believe. Yet it is entirely true. The vet who was on duty and dealt with the case (and I shall not disclose his identity) has recounted the story many times over the years.

The phone went early on the evening of 31 December.

'Hello, is that the vet?'

'Yes, what's the problem?'

'It's our cat. She's not very well,' explained the man on the end of the phone. 'We'd like you to have a look at her.'

'Okay,' replied my colleague, who was at home at the time. 'I can be at the practice in about ten minutes.'

It is always good to have a little bit of information, to be forewarned about what might be in store, so another tentative question followed, the answer to the first question not having been so illuminating.

'What has happened?'

'Well. We were bathing her in the sink — she was smelly, you see — and now she's not very well,' came the reply, which was still not that helpful.

'Okay, well I'll see you at the practice. If I'm not there immediately, just wait in the car and I'll be with you shortly.'

The unfortunate veterinary surgeon still didn't really know what the problem was, other than that the cat had been in the sink. He expected it to be wet.

When he arrived at the practice, the owners of the cat were already there, waiting in their car as instructed, clutching a large pink towel, swaddling the wet cat. He unlocked the front door and ushered them inside. People kept coming — it seemed it was a large family, and the small consulting room was filled with six quite large family members, who all gathered around the bundle on the table.

'So, tell me again what exactly happened this evening?'

It was important to know the full history. Animals (obviously) can't tell us vets the nature of their problem, so getting as much information as possible from owners is an important part of any assessment, even before the examination starts.

'Well, she was starting to smell, you see, so we thought we'd give her a bath. We bathed her in the sink in the kitchen and then . . . '

There was a pause accompanied by some snuffling from the youngest member of the group.

'And then she wasn't very well at all.'

It was becoming evident that a detailed history was not going to be forthcoming.

'Okay then, why don't we have a look — can you open up the towel please?'

The large pink towel was unravelled, to reveal a dead cat. A very dead cat. Rigor mortis had set in and it was completely stiff, with staring eyes and legs that stuck out rigidly.

The family stared expectantly at the veterinary surgeon for some kind of assessment of the sick tortoiseshell. Although there was clearly no need to listen for a heartbeat with the stethoscope, this seemed to be the only thing to do. After a few moments with the metal end resting on the cat's chest, the duty vet sadly shook his head.

'I'm sorry. She's passed away,' he said, confirming the obvious.

'Oh my God! She's DEAD?' was the collective response from all six members of the family. There was much wailing and grief, unsurprisingly as she was clearly a much-loved family pet. What was surprising was that nobody seemed to have had any clue that this might have been the case.

The family had a moment or two with their cat before wending a tearful way back home. Not a happy way to end the year, but a most unusual one. The most peculiar thought though, was that if they had embarked on the bathing process because the cat was starting to smell, and rigor mortis was well and truly established, how long had the cat actually been dead?

I don't think we'll ever know!

While You're Here . . .

Jobs like routine pregnancy tests, kennel inspections, calving cows or rescuing swans (or indeed establishing that an animal is dead) are all clearly defined tasks. We know exactly what the visit will entail and approximately how long it will take. Even though there are likely to be plenty of surprises along the way, once we have finished, the end point is clear. When the swan is caught and treated, or when the final cow has been tested, I can say 'cheerio', get back to the warmth of my car and go on to the next call. However, there is a certain phrase, usually uttered just as we are heading to the tap to wash off our wellies, which makes the heart sink. The farmer, almost accidentally, drops out the words:

'Ah, while you're here, Vet'nary, you couldn't just have a quick look at my . . .'

What comes next can be pretty much anything from ' . . . mother's elderly cat', to ' . . . heifer which has been slowly deteriorating from a chronic, obscure and impossible-to-diagnose disease (which happens to be still out in the field and on the other side of the valley)', or ' . . . yearling thoroughbred which I haven't been able to put a head collar on since I bought him three weeks ago'.

Whatever the nature of the 'while you're here' job, it is certain to mean that your carefully planned round of morning visits will overrun into lunchtime. It also means that lunchtime will cease to exist and morning visits will merge seamlessly into afternoon surgery. These 'while you're here' jobs are never announced before-hand and never discussed on arrival at the farm. No, this would be far too obvious. Everyone knows that we vets would rather have semi-urgent cases presented to us without warning, ideally at the last minute, just to keep us on our toes. It would never do if life were made too easy.

The master of the 'while you're here' job was Ray. He was farm manager at my favourite farm, on the edge of the North York Moors, halfway between Thirsk and Stokesley. It was a mixed farm, comprising a beef suckler herd of about one hundred adult cattle and follow-on stock, plus about two thousand sheep. In the early days of my time at Thirsk the farm also kept several hundred pigs. Add to this a heady collection of spaniels, the miscellaneous collies that always coexist with sheep and a few horses or ponies and the only certainty about any visit to this farm was that there would be more to do than you expected. What was uncertain though, was how many extras would be presented and of which species. Every visit would be like a kind of veterinary school final exam, where multiple different cases were paraded in front of me for diagnosis. The farm operated about six different units, which were spread over about three or four miles. Therefore, it was not uncommon to have a 'while you're here' job that wasn't 'here' at all. When Ray called the practice for a visit to see a

41

sick cow, you knew you would be there for the whole morning.

However, it still came as a surprise when all of the 'while you're here' jobs turned out to be on the same cow. It was late one evening when the call came in to visit the cow that, by strange misfortune, had managed to skewer itself on a big metal spike. This was particularly unlucky, because accidents of this nature usually happen on the most disorganised farms, where equipment is left pointing in all directions and the farmyard looks more like a junkyard. This was not the case here — the yard was impeccably well organised and very tidy. The spike in question was attached to the front of a tractor and used to carry large bales of hay, straw or silage. When not in use the spikes were left pointing to the ground to avoid injury to cows or people. However, the cow, heavy and heavily in calf, was lying down near the tractor and must have rolled under the spike, and then tried to get up, impaling herself through the right flank, with the spike advancing towards her lungs.

After some sedative and the injection of some local anaesthetic, it was possible to pull the metal spike carefully out of the cow. Mercifully it had missed the lungs. I spent some time cleaning the area and flushing the lengthy hole that extended deep into her abdomen. Luckily, the spike was clean and sharp and no pieces could have fallen off to become lodged inside the cow. This can, and often does, happen when the offending foreign body is a stick or a piece of wood and the outcome of such injuries is always very serious.

At least this wasn't the case tonight, and once I was happy everything was as clean as it could be, I set about suturing the injury back together. It took a while to repair and, as I got close to the end of the suturing, the cow lay flat on her side and started straining. Her eyes bulged and she began to make great bellowing and mooing noises. She was starting to calve.

Being a vet on a farm when an animal starts to give birth brings a certain responsibility. Whilst it is always best to allow things to take their natural course, it is folly to leave a calving cow, only to have to return two hours later, because she is having difficulty. So, having cleared away my surgical kit, I brought out the obstetrical lubricant. Lo and behold, when I reached inside to feel for the calf, all I could feel was its tail, and nothing else. This is the classic breech presentation. The calf is pointing backwards but with both back legs tucked forwards, towards the cow's head. It is impossible for the calf to be delivered naturally in this presentation, so intervention is always required.

There was nothing for it but to clean the blood from the first operation off my hands, and get an epidural ready. An epidural is essential when some serious rearrangement of the calf is required. It stops the cow from straining and therefore makes it possible to push the calf's bottom further in, allowing more space to manoeuvre its back legs up and back. It sounds rather grand when we announce that we will perform an epidural but it is actually a simple procedure, whereby about five millilitres of local anaesthetic solution is injected into the spinal cord, at the point where the tail joins the body. It numbs the whole area around the back of the cow, not only stopping her from straining, but also affording some pain relief during and after the delivery.

Even after the epidural injection had done its work, it took some huffing and puffing from me before the two back legs were eventually in the correct position, pointing backwards towards the way out. I attached a rope to each leg and, with the help of a calving jack (a ratcheted device that allows an even and continuous pull to be applied to the calf), the calf slowly emerged into the cold, dark world of North Yorkshire on this wintery night. When calves come out forwards their eyes are open, and they peer around as they slowly emerge and slither to the ground. I always think this gives them a few moments to get used to their new surroundings. But a backwards calf does not get this luxury. Once everything is lined up, you have to get them out quickly, because there is every chance the umbilical cord will break before the head is out, and the calf will take its first breath while still in the birth canal, where instead of air, it could inhale a lungful of amniotic fluid. So, I always feel slightly sorry for them as they land with a 'plop' on the ground. It must be quite a surprise.

This calf, though surprised, was very healthy and had survived both the trials of its mother being spiked and a difficult, breech delivery. It looked well, as did the weary cow. Ray and I congratulated ourselves on two good jobs in one

44

evening, and I began to think of a warm bucket of water to get cleaned up with before heading home. But this was not to be, because the cow had one final 'while you're here' job to throw at us, as she calmly and serenely prolapsed her uterus.

The uterus of a cow is a very large thing. Moments before, it was enclosing and nourishing the calf, which was now wriggling around on the straw, looking for a teat to suckle. With one not particularly big push from the cow, the whole uterus turned inside out and appeared, hanging from the back of her body. It was about the size and weight of a large sack of potatoes but in angry shades of red and purple, with mango-sized swellings all over its outer surface where the placenta had been attached. This was another emergency.

A uterine prolapse (or, as the farmers call it, a 'calf bed out') is very serious, and must be replaced as soon as possible. The cow can easily die of shock, sepsis or peritonitis if the uterus tears. I have seen cows charging around a cow shed with the whole lot hanging out, wobbling and swinging all over the place, the delicate tissue covered in straw and muck. Sometimes the cow can even stand on it with her hind feet. Cases like this usually go one of two ways — either they are quite easy to replace, slipping back in without too much problem, or they are extremely difficult: the friable uterine lining bleeds and ruptures as you handle it, and the outcome is not a happy one.

At least this time I was on hand at the very

moment it slid out, so there wasn't time for the uterus to become swollen and dirty. Despite all its misfortune, at least the cow had the luxury of the vet being right there, and she would have the most promptly replaced uterine prolapse ever! I felt optimistic that it would go well, for despite the cow being on its third major life-threatening event in the space of an hour and a half, I was fairly sure this one would be easily remedied. The odds were in her and my favour. Or so I thought.

However, as it turned out, the calf bed was very difficult to replace, as the uterine lining was fragile and prone to tearing when I touched it. After many painstaking minutes, it popped back inside and I managed to invert it completely. The last job was to place some nylon tape sutures in the vulva to stop the whole thing falling out again. Thankfully the epidural was still in action, so despite the rather sturdy needle required to do this, she didn't feel a thing.

Finally, I sat back on the bale of straw next to me and took a very deep breath, if not a sigh of relief. Surely my night's work was complete. Three procedures on one cow, all in the same night, was a most unusual event, and both Ray and I felt that she must now be well and truly sorted. I didn't linger on the bale for long, because she still needed a couple of injections before I could finally bid her, the calf and Ray good night — antibiotics to stop the otherwise inevitable infection, and pain relief, because goodness knows how much pain she must have been feeling. I shuffled back to my car boot to

46

get the required medication. On my return, and to my horror, the poor cow suddenly looked terrible. Her head stretched skywards and she let out an enormous 'Mooo'. Then she collapsed onto her side, took one last gasp and promptly died. The multitude of serious problems, one after another, was just too much for the poor cow's system.

★ ★ ★

Ray has retired now, but we still regularly attend the farm. John, the farm owner, who has taken over the running of the farm from Ray, called me out recently to see a cow he described, somewhat unusually, as 'lugubrious'. It was 'just not right'. This didn't really offer any clue as to the nature of the problem. The old phrase 'if only they could talk' is the perfect assessment of these situations. If only our four-legged patients could explain which bit was hurting — 'it's this bit just under my ribs', or 'there's a terrible burning pain in my bladder', or even 'I've got a splitting headache' — the job of a veterinary surgeon would often be easier. A lugubrious cow was a diagnostic challenge if ever there was one.

As I rolled up to the farm on this wet and miserable December morning I was unsure exactly what I would find. I quizzed John on the usual things — appetite, calving history, peculiar behaviour? Had there been any recent change in housing or diet? Were any other cattle affected? No — nothing to give me even the smallest clue. The group had been housed for a couple of

47

months and their silage diet was just the same. The cow was in good condition but had started to look poorly a few days previously.

I could see she looked uncomfortable. Her rumen was not contracting properly. Her temperature was just above normal — 102.5°F, not especially high, just up a bit. Her eyes were 'starey', which is a rather non-specific description, but to those experienced in peering at cows, it often points towards pain somewhere.

'Where does it hurt, old girl?' I wanted to ask.

Her lungs sounded clear, but as soon as I listened to her heart, the cause of the problem became apparent. The normal, steady 'lubb-dubb' beat was obscured by loud bubbling, squeaking and gurgling, characteristic of a serious condition called traumatic reticuloperi-carditis.

It all made sense. Her rumen would stop its regular waves of contraction with this condition, and she would be in considerable abdominal pain. A cow has four chambers to its stomach, and the first one, called the reticulum, sits just behind the diaphragm — a thin muscular sheet that separates the chest from the abdomen. On the other side of the diaphragm is the heart. Cows are not very tidy grazers — they tend to hoover up anything in their path. Sharp bits of wire, from fencing or from the inside of the tractor tyres used to weigh down the plastic sheets on top of the silage, tend to settle out in the bottom of the reticulum. This wire, if it is spiky enough, can pierce the diaphragm and, in extreme cases, penetrate the heart. Infection gets

48

in, and the sac surrounding the heart, called the pericardium, fills with thick pus. It makes the cow very poorly, it is very painful and it makes the heart sound like some sort of plumbing accident. This was exactly what I could hear. With the previous spike-related incident in mind, I quizzed John about any wire that could have got onto the grass or into the silage.

'We don't have any barbed wire on the farm,' John assured me, 'and we only use wrapped silage so we don't have old tyres.'

This was not what I wanted to hear as it spoiled my confident, although quite unusual, diagnosis. John looked unconvinced, but I assured him that this was *the* most likely situation, and that we needed to operate to avoid the inevitable demise of the cow. Even if we did operate, the prognosis would be grave, but at least she would have a chance. John knew me well and was accustomed to my occasionally wayward thought processes, so he agreed to the operation with only a little persuasion.

'Well, if that's what you think, we haven't got many options, have we? You'd better get on with it!'

And with that, he went to the tap to fetch two buckets of clean, warm water.

She was a big cow, and it was a long way down from where I would make my incision on her left flank to the base of her heart. Despite the cold and damp, there was nothing for it but to brave the chill and take off my shirt — I needed every bit of reach I could summon up, if I was right and there was a wire stuck through her diaphragm into her chest.

I clipped away some hair, scrubbed the skin and injected some local anaesthetic, then made a twenty-centimetre-long vertical incision on the cow's left side. Once I had gone through the skin, I cut through into the rumen. The rumen is basically a huge fermentation vat, where the indigestible fibre in grass, hay and silage is broken down into useful nutrients by millions upon millions of micro-organisms. It is a special smell that emanates from a rumen, and one that lingers for days. I needed to reach through eighty litres of fermenting grass soup, right to the bottom and right to the front, into the reticulum, to feel for the wire that I was hoping to find.

After not much exploring, I found a large and contorted piece of rope. It was a halter. This was not what I expected but, whilst it was not supposed to be there, I didn't think it was the cause of the problem.

'I haven't seen that halter for months!' spluttered John in astonishment. 'I thought one of you vets had driven off with it!'

I delved deeper, and suddenly, at the tips of my fingers, I could feel something hard. It felt like the head of a nail. I stretched as far as I could, wishing I had slightly longer arms. With my face jammed right up against the cow's side, I managed to pinch it between my finger and thumb. I didn't want to lose it. I pulled gently and the cow let out a grunt and jumped slightly. Like a magician pulling a rabbit out of his hat, I pulled my arm out, clutching in my hand a clean, shiny and very sharp four-inch nail!

There were gasps from John and his assistant Steven, who had arrived to watch.

'Bloody hell!' exclaimed Steven. 'That is amazing!'

Then, from John: 'That's a brand-new nail. Keep that, Steven, we can use it for the fencing work next week.'

There spoke a true Yorkshire farmer, I thought.

Billy and Betty

Mrs Taylor was a regular visitor to the surgery with her dogs, Billy and Mitzi. Billy was a shih-tzu, and ten years old. At least according to our records he was ten years old. Mrs Taylor had no idea how old he was. 'I think he's six,' she would declare confidently, despite computer evidence to the contrary. Mitzi was many years older than Billy, but even at the ripe old age of sixteen, the little black miniature poodle had boundless energy, and would constantly jump up and down, looking for anybody who would play with her. She was a live wire and full of fun. Billy, on the other hand, even though he was younger and fit and healthy, always had a 'hangdog' expression. Even when his tail wagged, it seemed that he was carrying the weight of the world on his canine shoulders.

I had known Mrs Taylor for many years. Before she had the companionship of these two little dogs, she and her late husband, Derek, had a jolly Staffordshire bull terrier called Butch. Staffies do not enjoy the best of reputations amongst the dog breeds, but they are in fact lovely dogs. Butch had a typically wide mouth, which made him look as if he were grinning from ear to ear. He had a tummy as round as Mr Taylor's, and his love for Derek was outweighed only by his dislike of the neighbour's cat.

The stout Staffy suffered from diabetes. His treatment involved daily injections of insulin and adherence to a strict diet. After weeks of adjustment and readjustment of his dose of insulin, Butch's blood sugar levels remained stubbornly high. I just could not get the diabetes under control.

Derek brought Butch in to the clinic every week, for me to check his blood and urine. The pair always sat, inseparable, in the same spot in the waiting room. Butch loved his visits, happily panting and watching all the other patients come and go, while Derek clutched his jam jar of frothy, yellow urine, in much the same way that a regular at the local pub would sit, nursing his pint in his usual spot. Derek was excellent at catching urine from his dog, even though there was not much space under Butch's tummy to fit a jam jar. He always provided an enormous sample. Only a few drops were actually required, but Derek took his job seriously.

'It's still high, I'm afraid, Mr Taylor,' I would explain as the bottom square on the urine dipstick changed to dark brown instead of the duck-egg blue that indicated a clear result. Derek was getting used to this news.

'Oh dear! Not again! Are we ever going to get this damn sugar under control?'

His accusatory tone suggested he thought it was my fault, maybe for not giving the correct type of insulin, or advising on the wrong dose.

'Are you *absolutely sure* you are injecting the stuff correctly?' I asked.

'Yes, of course I am! How difficult is it, after all?' came the reply.

'And you are keeping it in the fridge?'

No reply this time, just a vigorous nodding of the head.

'Butch is definitely just getting the food that we suggested, Mr Taylor?' There had to be a reason for the sugar level still being so high.

'Oh yes, of course! It's blooming expensive is that food — do you think I'd let it go to waste? I'm a pensioner, you know, I wouldn't waste good food,' came his rather defensive reply.

'Okay. We'll have to increase the dose of the insulin again. Up by another three units each time and then we'll have another sample in a week, if that's okay?'

I waved the happy dog and rather disgruntled owner goodbye, hoping that a bigger dose of insulin would do the trick. I wasn't completely confident that it would work. If we couldn't get the blood glucose levels down with this increase, I would need to do more tests. Maybe there was another condition, running alongside the diabetes, that was making Butch's body unresponsive to the insulin. But more blood tests would mean more expense, and I knew this wouldn't go down well with the pensioner.

The following week, Butch and Derek were back, sitting in their usual place. Derek grasped his jar of urine while Butch grinned at all the cats, lined up in their boxes, and tried to make friends with the other dogs in the waiting room. Next to Butch was an elderly lady, who I presumed to be Mrs Taylor.

I called them through, as usual, and Butch careered left and right down the waiting room, sniffing and smiling at all the other patients, who were waiting their turn.

'There you are,' Derek grumbled as he plonked his jar on the consulting room table. 'Let's hope we're on track this time! Oh, and this is my wife, Betty', he continued, as if it were an afterthought and of secondary importance to the delivery of Butch's urine.

'Thank you,' I said. 'Hello, Mrs Taylor. Nice to meet you.'

It was the first time we had met, as Butch was *Derek*'s dog and she did not take an active role in his treatment. I didn't imagine there was much discussion over dinner in the Taylor household about Butch's sugar levels.

I liked Mrs Taylor immediately. Some elderly ladies, with the advancement of years, lose their sense of humour in the presence of young vets ('How can this *very* young man possibly know how to treat my precious little cat? He looks barely old enough to be out of school!'), but I could tell by the glint in Mrs Taylor's eye that she definitely saw the funny side of life.

I dipped my urine test stick into the jar. It turned brown almost immediately — the glucose level was still very high. My heart sank. I was running out of ideas and I would need to do some blood tests today to check for additional problems.

By reflex alone, I repeated my usual diatribe of questions about extra food — maybe from next-door's bird table or a bowl of cat food?

Just as Derek was about to open his mouth in anger at my repeated questions, Mrs Taylor intervened.

'Oh yes, Derek feeds Butch all manner of sausage rolls and pork pies. Two or three times a day. Oh my, he does love them. I sometimes think old Butch will burst, he eats so many. Do you know, I'm not even sure whether it is Derek or Butch who eats more of them! They are a greedy pair, the two of them!'

It all started to make sense, but before I could make any comment and before Derek could offer his defence, Mrs Taylor was off again.

'That's why you're such a fat pudding, isn't it, Butchy boy?'

She patted the rotund terrier on the tummy and smiled at me, knowingly. I breathed a heavy sigh of relief. Finally, we had solved the mystery of the uncontrollable glucose levels.

'Well,' admitted Derek, 'I suppose he does get the odd one or two. He loves them, you see?'

I raised my eyebrows.

Once the pork pie situation had been rectified, Butch's health and waistline quickly returned to something like normal and I didn't see him so often at the practice, his blood sugar levels being finally sorted.

Some years later, both Butch and Derek had, sadly, passed away. I rarely saw Mrs Taylor, except for an occasional visit to clip the nails of her two guinea pigs, upon which she doted. She had acquired the two dogs, Billy and Mitzi, shortly after her husband had died but they didn't need a great deal of veterinary intervention. Both dogs were pretty healthy.

The problems with Billy began not long after Betty started getting weekly deliveries of frozen meals-on-wheels. Betty was baffled. She did not know why these meals kept appearing and she was certain she had no need for them. She knew what she liked and she knew how to cook. The pre-packed meals piled up in the freezer and the kitchen, and the obvious thing to do with them, as she saw it, was to heat them up and give them to Billy, who enjoyed them far more than he enjoyed his boring dog food. Billy was in danger of following in his predecessor's footsteps. He certainly loved the meals-on-wheels, but being a shih-tzu with a sensitive constitution, the result of this diet of roast dinners and toad in the hole was that Billy would often develop bouts of diarrhoea. This, in itself, was not particularly serious and it never affected Billy's ever-gloomy demeanour. However, the pasty, sticky consistency of the faeces meant that, once a little bit was glued onto his hairy bottom, it acted as a catalyst for more and more to become attached.

This was the problem that faced Billy (and me) when Mrs Taylor brought him to the surgery, one cold and gloomy November afternoon. Billy was a more reluctant patient than Butch had been. Mitzi ran in to greet me in the waiting room and then scuttled back to see Billy and Betty. She ran backwards and forwards several times as Billy, on his lead, made very steady progress towards the consulting room. At the last moment, he put on the brakes and sat down. Betty continued walking, unaware that her little dog had stopped, and Billy slid slowly along behind her, leaving a long stain as his dirty bottom smeared along the floor.

Finally, both dogs and Betty were in the room and the door was safely closed.

'Hello, Mrs Taylor. It's nice to see you. What can we do for Mitzi and Billy today?'

'Well, it's poo, poo, poo, poo, poo!' explained Betty. 'It's all under there!' She pointed under his tail. 'It's all STUCK there! I can't get it off. He's been in the shower and in the bath, but it's all STUCK ONTO HIM. Yuck!'

The problem was clear enough. I donned latex gloves and checked Billy all over, leaving his messy tail until the end of my examination. Despite his outward gloomy appearance, he was generally very healthy and I wasn't too concerned about that. It was the hairiness of his bottom, the stickiness of his poo and the difficulty that Mrs Taylor was having in cleaning him that seemed to be the predominant issues.

I explained what was needed. I would take Billy into the kennels, soak off the poo, clip the hair off his backside and give him a bath. Soon, he would be clean and happy. I set about the task with gusto. Many vets would have passed this job to a nurse, but I loved this sort of thing. The results would be instant and Billy would very quickly feel much better. It is not a glamorous job, but somehow it is very satisfying.

As predicted, within half an hour, Billy was rushing back to see Mrs Taylor, with infinitely more vigour.

'Oh Billy!' Betty exclaimed. 'You *are* lovely! What a lovely bum!'

I could think of nothing more to add.

Mitzi was still jumping up and down. I

thought she had just come along for the ride, but no. She was covered in warty spots, which Mrs Taylor was finding irksome.

'I keep catching them on my comb, you know, when I'm brushing her. Can you take them all off?'

It seemed a big job for an elderly dog. None of the warts carried a serious prognosis and they were certainly benign. However, Mrs Taylor was determined that I should remove them. I agreed, but arranged for her to come in another day — I hadn't expected that this appointment would take so long. It had been long-winded but very entertaining.

Two weeks later, Mitzi's warts had been removed and it was time to take her stitches out. Betty telephoned to explain that her car had been taken to the garage and she couldn't come to the practice. She asked if I could visit. Since the day was relatively quiet, and knowing that Betty was alone and would probably enjoy the company, I agreed to call round, on my way home for lunch.

When I arrived, Billy was relaxing on a cushion, looking out of the window. He leapt up and barked loudly as I came through the front door. Mitzi, who was deaf, only realized something was happening when she saw Billy become animated. At this point, she resumed her usual bouncing behaviour. It was difficult to keep her still as I removed the stitches, which were dotted about all over her body. I thought this was all I had to do, but Mrs Taylor had one more job for me.

'Do you know anything about televisions?' she asked. 'I can't make this thing work at all!'

The television was stuck on the Al Jazeera channel. It had been like this for the last week, according to Betty. She had been watching it anyway.

'I just can't work it out and I can't even understand what they are saying!' she laughed.

Once she started laughing it was hard not to laugh too, and soon we were both in hysterics at the whole situation — a dog with a newly trimmed bottom, a geriatric poodle who wouldn't stop bouncing up and down and a television that was broadcasting foreign news in a foreign language, which neither of us could understand or fix.

★ ★ ★

A few weeks passed. All three of the Taylor family had been healthy for a while. When I saw Billy's name on my morning appointment list, I presumed it was a return of his 'poo, poo, poo, poo, poo' problem, but Betty looked anxious. Mitzi burst into the consulting room as she always did, followed by Betty with Billy bringing up the rear.

'Is it the usual, Mrs Taylor?' I enquired.

'Julian. I'm very worried about Billy.'

He looked the same as ever to me. He sat gazing around benignly on the examination table, considering routes of escape — if only he had the energy.

'I've discovered a lump. It's under his tummy

60

and I think it's cancer'. Betty looked distraught.

'Okay, let's have a look. Whereabouts is it?' I asked.

'It's under his tum. Right under there, growing out of his skin.'

It wasn't immediately obvious where the lump was. I peered under his belly, around the soft part of his abdomen and around his ribs. These were the usual places for skin tumours to grow on a dog, but I couldn't find anything.

'It's underneath,' Betty explained, 'and I just noticed it today. It's very hard and I think it has grown very quickly'.

These were all features of an aggressive tumour. Poor Billy, he didn't deserve a serious tumour on top of his sensitive bowels.

Finally, I found the rock-hard mass, attached to the middle of his chest, right over his breastbone. Hard lumps like this are often aggressive sarcoma-type tumours originating from the hard connective tissue of the body. It felt about three centimetres long and about two centimetres across and was covered in sticky hair. This suggested the lump was discharging fluid. If a lump is oozing, the surrounding hair clumps and sticks to it in a tangled mass.

'It doesn't look very good I'm afraid, Betty.' I agreed with her suspicion that the lump could well be cancer.

'Ah, poor Billy!' She tried to reassure the worried dog as she stroked his fluffy head.

I decided to snip away some of the hair, to make it easier to see the lump underneath. After a few snips, I noticed a sticky feel to my fingers.

This lump had a very strange type of discharge. I was becoming more and more convinced it was going to be something really nasty. Then I noticed a distinctive minty smell emanating from the lump. The sticky appearance and minty aroma quite quickly changed my gloomy outlook to one altogether more positive.

'Mrs Taylor, I think it's a sweet!' I proclaimed with a grin. 'It's just a mint, I reckon. Billy has sat on a sticky mint and it has glued itself to his fur. It's not a tumour after all!'

It was hard to say who was more relieved.

'Oh Billy! It's a sweetie. It is. Oh Billy. A sweetie, stuck under his tummy!'

At which point, Betty and I both fell around laughing. It was the second time in a month.

'Well, Betty, I'd have felt a complete idiot if I'd put him under anaesthetic only to surgically remove a sweet!'

For a second time too, Billy's problem had been cured, not by tablets or surgical skill, but by my trusty scissors!

Our Lad and Our Lad

Away from the moors and towards the Vale of York, where the River Swale meandered its way towards the Ouse and then the Humber, and where a damp coldness persisted all winter, there was a dairy farm run by two brothers. When I first started work at Thirsk, I would visit every week or so because, although the farm was very well run, they had a steady stream of minor problems and were very keen on calling the vet to check that everything was in order with their stock. The damp air associated with the nearby River Swale seemed to bring a fair share of health issues to the herd, ranging from pneumonia in the young stock to problems in adult cows such as mastitis and lameness.

The brothers didn't get on, and they avoided conversation with one another at all costs. One brother would call the vet to see a cow or a calf that was sick, but would never dream of mentioning it to his sibling. When I arrived to see the case in question, the other brother would always be surprised to see me, but taking advantage of this serendipitous event, would rush off excitedly to get a completely different cow out of a field for me to examine.

The herd was medium sized, with about eighty cows, all of which were milked in a side-by-side milking parlour. This type of parlour, although quite old-fashioned, was commonplace in Thirsk

63

at that time. It allowed about eight cows to be milked together, standing in pairs next to each other. The cows stood up on a concrete step about half a metre high. This allowed the farmer to attach the milking cluster to the udder, without bending down too far and thus saving his back from extra wear and tear. However, for the vet, it made the job of carrying out an examination per rectum completely impossible without something to stand on. During a fertility visit to a dairy farm that used this system, the most critical piece of equipment was not a scanner, a rectal glove, or a bottle of 'lube', but a plastic box to use as a stool.

The thing that amused me about visits to this farm was the way the two brothers referred to one another. They both called the other one 'Our Lad'. It was not particularly unusual in this part of the world for siblings to refer to each other by this affectionate term, but here they also used it when talking about the other brother to a third party, such as me, and very little affection was involved. It became quite confusing, trying to work out who was talking about whom, and to whom. At times, I thought I should just join in and call them both by the same name, 'Our Lad'.

The only time I heard them addressed by their real names was by their mother, when she emerged from the farmhouse with a tray of hot drinks, or to mediate in an argument between the two of them about the course of treatment for a cow.

One wintery day, with frozen fog hanging low

in all the hollows, I was called by Our Lad to visit some sick calves. Days like these are beautiful, especially when the watery winter sun is out, and only the tops of the trees emerge from the wispy low fog. My car tyres cracked the ice that was covering the many puddles on the track to the farm. The calves were suffering from a nasty condition called 'scour', which is the colloquial term for diarrhoea. It is fairly common in young cattle during winter. In these short, dark days when cattle are inside to protect them from the cold and bad weather, they are in greater contact with one another than when they are out at grass. They are also usually on deep beds, kept clean by adding new straw on top, which is very warm and cosy, but does result in an increased chance of infection. The incidence of scour rises as winter progresses but, once animals go back out to the fields in spring, the likelihood of this disease usually dissipates. Today, Our Lad was understandably quite worried. Meanwhile, his brother, Our Lad, was not at all worried. He was more involved with the older cattle, and obviously they would never discuss an emerging problem between themselves before I arrived.

I checked the calves and took the necessary samples to drop off at the lab on the way back to the practice. In those days, there was a VIC (Veterinary Investigation Centre) in Thirsk to deal with this sort of thing. It was fantastic to be able to call in, drop samples off in person and speak, face to face, with the experts who worked there. These labs were run by MAFF (the

Ministry of Agriculture, Fisheries and Food), now known as DEFRA (the Department for Environment, Food and Rural Affairs), and were (and still are) critical in disease control in food-producing animals. Nowadays though, due to government cuts and restructuring (more cuts), the lab is on its last legs and barely does any testing at all. Today we are reprimanded for delivering samples in person, because it contravenes the regulations.

The calves looked poorly. They all had high temperatures. Most of them were very, very loose and some were actually passing blood. I immediately suspected salmonella as the cause. The faeces test would tell me the answer, but first I had to speak to the brothers together to explain my theory. If I was right, then there was a real risk to human health on the farm, as well as to all the stock. They would need a coordinated hygiene strategy, with disinfectant boot dips and thorough cleaning of kit, housing and people. In short, they would have to work together on this one.

After I had finished running through the hygiene rules I had enforced, pending results from the lab, there was a stony silence that seemed to last minutes.

The silence was broken by Our Lad.

'Okay, while you're here, Vet'nary, Our Lad has a cow for you to look at.'

I was only mildly surprised. I had already scrubbed and disinfected my wellies, to rid them of any salmonella bugs that might be lurking in the crevices after being in with the calves, but this was essential before going to see one of the adult cows anyway, as we didn't want to spread infection.

'Our Lad thinks this cow is a mad cow. Well, it's not a mad cow I'm sure, but Our Lad thinks it is,' said Our Lad.

'Okay, let's have a look,' I offered, trying to take a neutral position.

Cases of 'mad cow disease' were few and far between by this time, at the end of the 1990s. Most suspicious cases had been killed and incinerated so, in the early part of my veterinary career, as the BSE (bovine spongiform encephalopathy — the technical name for mad cow disease) crisis was reaching its end, I didn't see many. Our Lad and Our Lad, though, had both seen a few cases during those dark years, but although they were quite experienced at recognizing them, there was clearly some dispute today.

The 'mad' cow was standing in the collecting yard, shaking. I walked her around, to see how she moved. She walked in a twitchy, shaky way and was obviously unsteady and unsure on her feet. Some of this might have been due to the slippery ice on the ground, but I felt sure she was shaking more than she should have been, even given the treacherous terrain.

'Can we get her into a crush or a cubicle to examine her?'

I wanted to say 'Our Lad?' after this sentence, but it didn't seem the right thing. I need not have worried, because Our Lad had already sprung into action.

'Let's get her into the parlour.'

The trembling cow was persuaded into the parlour and up onto the concrete platform, where she would usually be milked. This was a big step for a shaking cow and the effort clearly took its toll, so that her whole head and ears were shaking as well as her body. I took my thermometer, stethoscope, rectal gloves and blood sample tubes so I could examine the cow properly and take the right samples. Given that one brother thought this cow had mad cow disease, and the other brother thought differently, my diagnosis would be more pressured than most.

She was showing many of the classic signs, but cases of BSE had declined dramatically over the recent months and I did not like to jump to this terrible conclusion. I came up with a plan that would, hopefully, lead me to the right diagnosis and at the same time placate the feuding brothers.

I explained what I had in mind. 'I'll get some blood samples to check for nervous ketosis and to see if her magnesium levels are okay.'

The faces of both brothers looked confused, as neither of them had heard of 'nervous ketosis' and didn't know why magnesium levels were relevant to this cow.

Nervous ketosis is a version of a condition called 'slow fever', with which both farmers were very familiar. It is a condition seen in cows shortly after they have calved, when the body tries to metabolize its fat reserves to provide energy. It comes about if the body's adjustment

68

to producing large volumes of lactose-rich milk is not a smooth one. The amount the cow can eat can't keep pace with the increased need for energy, and the result is that the body calls on its fat reserves. This works very well, up to a point, but if the demand is too high, it can lead to the build-up in the bloodstream of chemicals called ketones. Usually, this ketosis causes the cow to stop eating (the worst thing she could do at this point) and become dull and lethargic, but in severe cases they can develop crazy behaviour — madly twitching their ears and sometimes frantically licking metal gates and other strange things.

Magnesium deficiency usually leads to an acutely serious and often fatal condition called 'staggers'. The cow becomes wobbly (hence the name), then collapses, convulses and dies if she is not treated quickly. However, sometimes a cow can have a low-grade magnesium deficiency, which makes her tremble rather than convulse. It was a long shot, but worth checking, for thoroughness if nothing else and, although both 'Our Lads' looked unconvinced, it got me off the hook of coming down in favour of one sibling instead of the other.

I explained that I would take the blood samples to the lab, along with the faeces samples that I had collected from the calves. The results would be back within a couple of days, and should tell me everything I needed to know. If the samples from the shaking cow were negative for ketosis and the magnesium was normal, I would have to call the ministry to report it as a suspected case of BSE. It was their job to make the final decision.

I bade them both farewell, after another thorough cleaning under the tap with copious volumes of disinfectant. Luckily, my journey back to the practice took me right past the veterinary laboratory, where I called in to hand in the samples.

As I was filling in the required paperwork, I caught sight of the senior vet who worked at the lab. I attracted his attention and sought his advice on the shaking cow.

'Well, if you think it's BSE, don't talk to me about it! You need to speak to the Divisional Veterinary Manager at Leeds. Not my job, you know!'

I looked at him in disbelief, as he went on.

'I thought all you vets knew that the correct procedure is to report notifiable diseases to the DVM.'

And with that he was off. It was half past four in the afternoon, which was the time that ministry vets finished their day. There was no way he was hanging around to point any advice in my direction.

Disappointed by his lack of assistance, I completed my submission form and posted it through the window of the reception desk before negotiating the traffic through the twinkling lights of the early evening in Thirsk, back to the practice where evening surgery beckoned.

Two days later, the results came back. The calves, as I suspected, were positive for salmonella. The shaking cow, however, had neither chronic hypomagnesaemia nor nervous ketosis. I telephoned the farm to break the news. The salmonella result was bad — it was a serious disease and there was a grave outlook for the calves without some intensive treatment. But it was manageable with strict hygiene, appropriate antibiotics for the sick ones and vaccination for the rest of the herd.

In a way, though, the negative result for the shaky cow was worse, because it made a diagnosis of BSE more likely. I called the DVM straight away, as I had been instructed to do, but spoke to one of his deputies.

I explained the signs and the history.

'What you should do is test it for hypomag and ketosis,' said the duty vet on the end of the phone. 'It's very unlikely to be BSE. We haven't had a case of that for months now. The epidemic has passed and thank goodness for that. Terrible problem it was, wasn't it?'

I sighed and explained again that I had already ruled out the conditions he had mentioned. At this, his tone changed and he reluctantly agreed to arrange a visit to inspect the cow, as was the proper procedure. Only ministry vets were allowed to make the diagnosis of BSE.

I called Our Lad and Our Lad again to tell them that the ministry would be in contact soon to arrange a visit. I could hear the argument starting even before I had put down the telephone.

'I bloody told you it was mad cow!'

'I bloody told you it wouldn't be!'

At least this time, the responsibility of making the diagnosis and upsetting one or other Our Lad wouldn't fall to me.

A Leg at Each Corner

The note next to the appointment on the computer was clear enough:

Have told Mrs C that vet will not supervise a mating during afternoon surgery.

The following note, happily for me, passed the responsibility elsewhere:

See nurse.

I went in search of a nurse who might be able to help, although I was not confident I would find a willing volunteer. No one could offer any more details either.

'Well, the lady just said she was having trouble getting her bitch in pup, and she wanted you to check everything was all right.'

Not much the wiser, I set about the afternoon's appointments — the usual mix of boosters, itchy dogs, poorly cats and the odd rabbit. At three o'clock, there was a commotion in the waiting room. I poked my head round the consulting room door to see two slightly embarrassed dog owners standing at the reception desk. At their feet were two dogs. One was a little Yorkshire terrier, the other a somewhat stout Norfolk terrier. The Norfolk was doing his very best to mount the Yorkie, who was looking casually around the waiting room. She seemed rather bored.

'You had better come through,' I called, aware of the startled expressions on the faces of some of the other clients.

'How can I help?' (This was a redundant question, because I knew what the embarrassed owners expected, but I had to ask.)

'Well, we have been trying to get them to mate for the last two years, and it just doesn't seem to be working. We can't understand it. We hoped you could help?'

I looked at the two dogs. The bitch was clearly at the peak of her season and standing patiently, tail cocked helpfully to one side, while the sandy-coloured Norfolk terrier enthusiastically tried to do his thing. If the Yorkie had been human she would definitely have been sighing and rolling her eyes with frustrated disappointment.

'Have you tried her with a different dog?' I ventured.

'Oh no, we want puppies from these two — they will be perfect, just what we want. She is just so lovely, and he is such a character, and well, just think how cute their puppies will be . . .'

But the problem was abundantly clear after just the briefest of examinations. I wasn't sure how to break it to these two devoted owners. I couldn't quite believe they hadn't noticed.

Norfolk terriers are sturdy little dogs and this one was no exception. He was like a little round barrel with a short leg at each corner. He was doing his very best, but his tummy was in the way, and his legs weren't long enough. Neither was his penis. He just couldn't reach. There wasn't even anything particularly scientific I could say.

'I'm really sorry,' I said, cringing slightly. 'He isn't getting her in pup because his penis won't reach. Look — it's miles away!'

The two ladies stared at me in horror. I was having trouble keeping a straight face.

'Oh my goodness, you're right. What can we do?'

'Well, nothing really. Maybe you should give up on this match — they are both obviously very frustrated, and he isn't going to manage.'

Everyone gazed down at the two dogs, who were both oblivious to the fact they were in the veterinary surgery, and the subject of everyone's attention. They were both still vainly trying to do what nature didn't quite intend. There was a long silence. Clearly someone was waiting for me to come up with a miraculous solution.

'I know!' exclaimed Mrs C. 'Maybe we could stand him on something? Or pick him up — could you do that — pick him up so he can reach? Could we try that now?'

This didn't seem like a good idea at all — me standing there dangling a rotund terrier behind a bitch so they could have cute puppies. And all in the middle of afternoon surgery. I politely explained that if they couldn't mate naturally, it was probably best to abandon the idea altogether.

It took some persuasion, but eventually the

disappointed owners accepted that this, perhaps, wasn't the perfect union after all.

Imagine my surprise then, when some months later, when winter had worn into spring, the leaves had appeared on the trees and the dark nights were behind us for another year, Mrs C appeared in the waiting room with a scruffy, sandy-coloured puppy. I couldn't believe my eyes. Images of steps, boxes or hoists sprang to mind.

'Is that . . . ?'

She laughed.

'No, you were right about that! After we left you, I drove straight up to see my friend in the Dales. She has a Jack Russell. I opened the car door, and he was straight there — it only took two minutes!'

SPRING

As the days begin to lengthen and snowdrops optimistically make their appearance in the hedgerows of North Yorkshire, I get the first sense that the worst of winter is behind us. It is the beginning of the busiest and best time of the year for us at Skeldale. It is the start of lambing time. To anyone connected with sheep, 'lambing time' is a season all to itself, just as significant as springtime or summertime. It is all-consuming. Some farmers do not even go to bed during this period, but instead take short snatches of sleep in a chair in the kitchen between checks on the flock. These farmers get slowly more grey, more weak and more fragile as the weeks of lambing go on.

Lambing time is very intense and it has to be, because each mother and her offspring must be closely supervised and nurtured from birth to the time at which they are turned out onto the spring grass. If lambing were protracted over several months, as calving time often is for a beef herd, farmers would never be able to stay focused. A flock of up to a thousand sheep typically lambs over a period of about four weeks. The expectant mothers are brought indoors, or at least close to the farm and into shelter. Extra staff (often in the form of veterinary students) are drafted in to help cover night shifts and the multitude of tasks associated with lambing, such as bedding and feeding the expectant mothers. These are jobs that aren't required for most of the year, when ewes are pretty much self-sufficient in the pastures or on the hill.

Lambing ewes demand a high degree of supervision during labour. Lambs can vary tremendously in size, and some big ones will not make it to the outside world without a helping hand from a human. The most frequent problems, however, come about because lambs are often born in multiples — twins are the norm, but sometimes triplets and even quads. The lambs and their long limbs often get tangled into a jumbled mess inside the uterus, so that once the contractions start, different bits of different lambs are all squeezed into the birth canal at the same time. This demands intervention, either from an experienced farmer or a veterinary surgeon who can untangle the lambs and deliver them one by one. It is always a source of bafflement to an inexperienced lambing student when they are sure that a lamb is presented perfectly and yet still refusing to budge — because the legs and head they have carefully lined up are not from the same lamb!

Once the lambs have been delivered in a slippery heap onto the straw, shaking their heads and struggling to coordinate their legs, the work of the sheep farmer is only just beginning. The mother and babies need to be moved to an individual pen as soon as possible. Here they can form a close bond — one that will persist during their time together on the moor. The strength of this bond is critical to the health and welfare of the lambs, as they grow. Sheep breeds are selected specifically for the strength of their mothering instincts, but it is important to keep mother and babies together without distractions for a few days. Sheep are easily confused and the worst scene for a shepherd, on arrival at the lambing shed first thing in the morning, is a group of ewes, all of whom have lambed in close succession during the night, and who cannot decide whose lamb is whose. The lambs cannot fathom out which woolly milk bar belongs to them, and there is always one ewe who claims three lambs, while another, who has clearly given birth, doesn't want anything to do with any of them. Sadly, they don't come out with labels on.

That said, once the lambs have been licked clean by their mum, labelling them up is exactly the next job! Indelible marker spray has been a godsend to sheep farmers. It allows them to spray a number on the sides of both ewe and lambs, so they are permanently identified as a family, exactly like applying a band to the wrist of a newborn baby in a maternity hospital. With garishly bright numbers daubed on their sides, the sheep and lambs do not look quite so photogenic when they are skipping around in the bright green fields when proper spring arrives, but to the farmer, marking them like this makes life much easier. Ewes and lambs are matched up for good.

The new families stay in their individual pens until it is clear the lambs can suckle properly. Some are particularly dozy and it takes hours of supervision to get them going. Their navels are dipped in iodine to prevent infection, and the ewes are wormed, before they are moved into bigger pens of half a dozen ewes and lambs together. This is a great time for the lambs. They start to make their acquaintance with other lambs and the playing begins.

Lambing time is condensed into a period of a few weeks not just for the farmer's convenience, but because of the way that sheep breed naturally. Most native breeds of sheep come into season in the late summer or autumn, when the hormones that make this happen are triggered by the shorter day length. The ewes, therefore, all come into season at roughly the same time, at which point they are mixed with the tups (male sheep). Since the gestation period of a sheep is about one hundred and fifty days (around five months), ewes tupped in November will be due to lamb in April.

Some farmers choose to tup their ewes earlier in the year than at the end of summer. This is possible with some breeds. Lowland breeds such as the Suffolk come into season earlier, whereas upland breeds like the Swaledale, which have to lamb and survive in tougher conditions on the moors and hilltops of Yorkshire, do not naturally come into season until later in the autumn. This means that their lambs are (theoretically) born in more favourable weather conditions, later in the spring. Nature is clever like that. So, whilst each farm will have a closely defined lambing period dictated by the breed of sheep, in a veterinary practice like ours there will be sheep to lamb from the start of January to the end of April. Add to this the various pre-lambing problems and the multitude of post-lambing complications, and we spend about half of our year dealing with sheep and lambs and their health. This is a good thing though, because we all like working with sheep.

Lambs' Tales 1: Grange Farm

It was always fun going to lamb a sheep at Grange Farm. The farm was in Old Byland right on the top of the Hambleton Hills. Farms at the top of Sutton Bank are all made of stone blocks, rather than the orangey-red narrow bricks of lower-lying farms. The farmhouse was always an impressive sight as I drove up the sweeping track to the entrance.

The farm belonged to two sisters, Doreen and Kathleen, and their brother Brian. They kept cattle and sheep, and reared turkeys and geese for Christmas. It was part of our family Christmas ritual for my sons and me to go up to Grange Farm, the day before Christmas Eve, to collect a turkey. We would be welcomed into the stone-flagged farmhouse as the best of friends. The boys would be given wine gums to chew on, while I was offered cups of tea and Christmas cake. The kitchen was packed with almost all the locals, chatting and drinking tea as they each collected their own Christmas turkey or goose. The family was well regarded in the local community, not just because of their farming prowess, but also because they were kind folks, living a simple and straightforward life. It was the life of a disappearing era.

When I arrived to lamb a sheep, there would always be a bucket of warm water, a bar of soap and some clean towels at the ready. I would be ushered into the dark lambing shed, and given a brief and succinct assessment of the problem. As I rummaged around, trying to make sense of the legs and heads, Doreen would stare at me intently with her animated face, hanging on every word of my answer to the question she always asked, as I was midway through the job of lining up the lambs for delivery: 'Do you like lambing?'

She knew I did, because I always answered her question in the same way, every time I visited the farm for this particular job, or any other job, for that matter. We didn't have to lamb sheep at Grange Farm very often, as the siblings were skilled shepherds and rarely needed assistance, so it could have been that Doreen had forgotten my answer to her favourite question. But somehow, I doubted it.

On this particular day, as usual, I assured Doreen how much I *did* like lambing, but then she surprised me with another question, taking her usual interrogation to a new level.

'Do you think you are better or worse at lambing sheep than that 'Meechy Vet' who lives in Cold Kirby?'

I was somewhat thrown by this, since I had never been asked to compare my clinical skills with another professional before. I knew the 'Meechy Vet' well: Stewart Mechie lived in the next village to Doreen but had only recently started working with us at Skeldale. His lambing skills had not yet been tested on this farm and there was obviously some debate among the farming community about his capability, as if his reputation preceded him. I was sure he was excellent at lambing sheep, but I did not dare to compare myself.

So, to avoid direct comparison of our skills, I replied, 'Well, Doreen, I'm sure Stewart is a very capable lamber. He's from Scotland and he's done a lot of this sort of thing before. But really, I wouldn't like to say which of us is actually the best.'

Doreen promptly misinterpreted my tact and discretion. She thought I was trying to be modest and immediately presumed that I was quietly confirming that 'yes, the 'Meechy Vet' is indeed a good lamber, but not *quite* as good as I am!'

Gasps and exclamations came from Doreen, as if she were the first to learn the exciting news of a ranking amongst the vets at Skeldale! I tried to protest and reaffirm that I really didn't know which of us was the best at lambing sheep and that it really didn't matter too much anyway. But it fell on deaf ears. The more I tried to clarify the situation, the bigger the hole became that I had dug for myself.

Doreen realized she had hit on a potential controversy and continued gleefully. 'And what about Peter? He likes lambing.' (He had been questioned about this many times more than I had and Doreen had obviously not forgotten this.) 'Would you say you are better or worse at lambing than *him*?'

And so the questions continued, listing all vets in the practice, both present and past. I quickly gave up my initial plan of remaining noncommittal and fell in line, providing Doreen with all the information she needed to decide who was the best. I could only imagine the rumour and conjecture that would spread around this part of Ryedale when Doreen went on her weekly shopping trip to the local town of Helmsley a few days later.

I was in an inescapable situation. I had finished delivering two healthy lambs several minutes previously (I was, after all, an excellent lamber — if not *the* best), and was now cleaning my hands and my wellies, but it seemed the only way to finish the discussion was to agree with Doreen and her ranking system.

As I collected the swedes that Doreen's brother Brian had, as usual, produced for me to take home ('Do you like swedes?' was his favourite parting question), I pondered the long-term implications of our discussion.

In years to come, every time a challenging lambing came in from Grange Farm, the message in the daybook would say:

Bentley — Grange Farm, Old Byland.
Visit: ewe to lamb. Very difficult.
JN if possible.

Lambs' Tales 2: Balk Beck

My impeccable reputation at Grange Farm did not extend to all the farms looked after by the practice. Alf Wight, better known to the animal-loving world as James Herriot, had a phrase that all enthusiastic veterinary surgeons would be wise to remember: 'You are only as good as your last job.'

Farmers around Thirsk, and probably everywhere else too, have long memories when things don't go according to plan, but often quite short memories when it comes to stories of success on their farm. A hard-earned reputation can easily be blown away by a bad decision whilst calving a cow, or the wrong choice of drugs to treat a calf with a severe case of pneumonia.

There is one farm where, if father and son were following Doreen's ranking system, I would certainly be at or somewhere very close to the bottom.

I had been called to see a heavily pregnant ewe. She had fallen into a stream, swollen by heavy springtime rain. The stream, 'Balk Beck', which on this day was more like 'Balk River', ran right through the middle of the farmyard and separated the farmhouse from most of the farm buildings, which were reached via a little bridge. In days past, there was a watermill on the farm. It would harness the power of the gently flowing stream to grind grain and turn it into flour. The days of the watermill were long gone, but Balk Beck was still a significant feature of the farm.

This spring, the beck had flooded, which caused problems for the in-lamb sheep grazing in the nearby paddock. It was knee deep in water. Most of the ewes had sensibly manoeuvred themselves to the edge of the field and were safe from the overflowing torrent, but my poor, waterlogged and weary patient was not so fortunate. She had been found bobbing about in an eddy current just downstream from the little bridge.

Sheep have a large rumen, half full of gas, so even though they are not very competent swimmers, they do float very well. Just like Eeyore in the famous Winnie the Pooh story, this sheep had obviously been bobbing around in the water for some time. By the time she had been scooped out of the stream by Mick and his son Andrew, all she could do was lie, flat and moribund, on her side in the soggy paddock. She couldn't walk and her waterlogged fleece made her too heavy to be carried. When I arrived, Mick and Andrew were standing next to her, in the place from where she had been fished out, with their hands on their hips. Strictly speaking, Mick only had one hand on his hip, since his right hand was occupied with his ever-present cigarette.

'Bah! She looks badly, Vet'nary,' he wheezed between puffs.

'I think she's abart buggered, Dad!' offered Andrew, in a typically astute and terse assessment of the situation.

'I think she is, son,' confirmed Mick, in a 'that's my lad' kind of way.

It seemed that both my services and my opinions were surplus to requirements, as the three of us stood and stared at the almost drowned ewe. I hadn't said anything useful so far and I had no specific remedy in my car boot to cure a hypothermic and waterlogged sheep. She was only marginally closer to life than she was to death. Then it occurred to me that we might be able to salvage something from the dire situation.

'Is she in lamb, Mick?'

'Aye, she's due next week by the look of her mark.'

All the sheep were marked with a spot of colourful dye on their backs, which showed when they had been mated by the ram. At tupping time, each ram would carry a raddle — a sort of harness, with a paint cartridge attached on the front. The farmer would change the colour on the raddle every week, so they could tell when the ewe had been mated by the colour on her back. In this way, an approximate lambing date could be calculated.

The poor ewe was fading fast, but I thought there was a possibility we could at least save the lambs, by performing a 'bush' caesarian. This is a way of saving the unborn lambs from a terminally ill sheep (or calf from a cow or foal from a mare). A quick and efficient caesarian section is performed before the dam is euthanased on humane grounds. Done correctly and at the right time, this can save the life of an unborn lamb in a situation where otherwise both mother and baby would perish.

I discussed the plan with Andrew and Mick, who seemed to think it was a good idea. They hadn't seen a caesarian before, and anything that would make an otherwise sad morning better was worth a go. I was somewhat pessimistic about the chance of success — experience had taught me that an emergency caesarian like this, on a sheep that was some way from its natural lambing date, was fraught with problems. The lambs only become mature enough to survive in the last few days of gestation, and by Mick's calculations, they weren't due for another week. Nonetheless, it was the only hope of some sort of positive outcome.

I got what I needed from the car and swiftly clipped away some soggy wool. I numbed the area with local anaesthetic, then got a syringe ready with the solution that I would use to euthanase the sheep after her lambs were out. I knew I had to be quick and time was of the essence. If the ewe were to beat me to it and die before I had delivered the lambs, their chances of survival would be even lower.

Sadly, this is exactly what happened and, only moments after the local had gone in, she took one last breath and promptly expired. Ever the optimist, I quickly whipped out my scalpel and made a swift and bold incision — hoping it might not be too late to save the lambs.

However, my incision was a bit too swift and a bit too bold. The puffy, oedematous skin and muscle were weaker than I expected, and my scalpel, in one sweep, went right through the skin, muscle and uterus. I pulled out the first lamb which I could instantly tell was more than a week premature. It was also very dead.

Mick and Andrew could not tell from their vantage point that the lamb was premature and dead, but they could tell quite quickly that my scalpel had made a long gash into its flesh.

'Bah! Vet's slashed lamb!' exclaimed Andrew at the top of his voice to his father.

I had, indeed, slashed the lamb, although this was entirely irrelevant to the lamb, since it had died several hours previously, presumably as the body systems of its mother were shutting down in the cold water of the river. I tried to explain, but my protestations fell on deaf ears.

Moments later, I felt somewhat redeemed, as I pulled out a second lamb. It was free from any kind of slash mark, but equally dead. Several hours of bobbing around in the cold water had obviously been too much for all concerned.

It seemed, though, that in the eyes of father and son, it was all my fault. As they splashed their away across the flooded paddock, I was certain I would never be allowed back onto the farm.

Poppy or Penny?

It doesn't always rain in springtime in Thirsk. As spring progresses, the wet and wintery weather eases into lighter nights and longer days. When there are emergency calls to do in the evening, some days are longer than others and one particular April day was longer than most.

It was about half past seven, at the end of a busy evening surgery. I was heading across the car park with the 'on-call kit' — a big box containing the calving jack and all the equipment needed for doing a caesarian on a cow (or any other large surgical procedure). I hadn't even got as far as my car before my beeper went off. Instead of locking up the surgery and heading home for tea, I went back inside to phone the answering service for details of the emergency.

The beeper message said there had been a road traffic accident on the A1 and my attendance was required immediately. These calls are always complicated. Not only is there an injured and terrified animal (or animals) to deal with, but there is the danger inherent with high-speed traffic whizzing past. Usually we have to coordinate with the traffic police to make things safe for everyone concerned.

A dog had been hit, reported the person at the answering service, and people were sitting with it on the hard shoulder. Could I go right away?

The accident was on the southbound carriageway of the A1, not far from Richmond. It was a long way away, some twenty miles outside our normal area. Calls like this are a tricky issue because our foremost responsibility is to our own clients, within our practice area. If I am tied up for most of the night somewhere miles away, it falls to the vet on second call to deal with all the other work that comes in during the evening. There were at least four other veterinary practices closer to hand than I was, but we did a lot of work for the police so were often their first port of call.

Despite these issues, the moment my beeper chirped into life, I felt I was responsible for the case. I gathered all the things I would need. Dogs that have been hit at high speed by a car are usually badly damaged and they can react in an aggressive way, for no other reason than being frightened and in great pain. One of my patients, a gentle and benign German shepherd dog called Jed, who belonged to Sue, a receptionist at the practice, was in such terrible pain after being hit by a car that when she tried to help him, the poor dog actually bit her finger off. This was not what I wanted tonight so, armed with medicines, bandages, blankets and a selection of muzzles, I clambered into the practice van/animal ambulance and set off.

As usual, there were major roadworks on the A1. As I got close to the site of the incident, I could see the commotion on the opposite side of the road. There was a traffic control vehicle and another car. I could see people sitting on the hard shoulder, but I had to drive further north for another ten minutes before I could get out of the roadworks and back down to the injured dog and its rescuers.

A bewildered, confused and seriously injured pointer bitch was swaddled in a fleece jacket belonging to the lady who was comforting her. Both of them, as well as the fleece, were covered in dark, congealed blood.

'Oh, thank goodness you're here!' said the lady, who introduced herself as Sheila. She was in almost as much of a state of shock as the poor dog.

'We were just driving along and right in front of us this dog ran out and straight under a lorry. It didn't even stop — it just carried on. We swerved and then stopped to pick her up, and stop her running into the road again. I wrapped her in this jumper and then I called you. I'm heading back to Rotherham and I'm really late already. We've been here for over an hour!'

Sheila had done a great job in catching and comforting the dog. I felt sure that, had she not stopped her car to help, the dog would have been hit a second time and would not have survived. Not only that — there could have been a serious accident. The dog wasn't wearing a collar so Sheila was keeping hold of her in an awkward hug. No collar meant no obvious owner to contact, and no indication of her name. It is always nice to be able to call a dog by its name.

I slipped a lead over the dog's head to make sure she didn't escape and then, mindful of the aforementioned finger incident, put a muzzle on

— just in case — as she was, no doubt, very frightened and in a great deal of pain. Then I examined her as best I could. She was concussed and there was bruising around her face and head. Her lungs sounded noisy, which was suggestive of bruising to this delicate part of the body, and could be serious. There was a large and painful swelling around the upper part of her left front leg. The telltale floppiness of the limb was a sure sign that there was something seriously wrong. It was either a broken humerus or a dislocated shoulder, both equally bad and equally painful. I needed to do some x-rays to establish the full extent of her injuries.

Without delay, I injected a dose of morphine into the muscle of her back leg. This would act quickly and effectively to take away much of the pain. It would also act as a sedative, so the journey to the surgery would be less stressful for her. I wrapped her in a blanket and gently lifted her out of Sheila's arms. There was no doubt that this dog would not have been alive had it not been for Sheila's help. Before she left with her bloodstained fleece, her face and clothes also all smeared with blood, she wrote down her telephone number so I could keep her updated on the dog's progress.

And with that, I headed back to the practice to work out what needed to be done. I stopped every so often to check on my patient. She was having a peaceful journey as the morphine took effect. In the absence of an actual name, I decided to call her Poppy, mainly because she was a pointer and I thought that a name beginning with the letter 'P' would be easy to remember. Poppy Pointer was the first thing I could think of and it seemed better to call her something rather than nothing. Even if it didn't bother the dog (being called by her correct name seemed the least of her worries), it made it easier for me.

Having returned to the surgery, my first job was to check for a microchip. With baited breath I pressed the 'on' button and the transceiver flickered into life. The single, jubilant 'BEEP' gave me the news that I wanted. The dog had a chip, which meant she had an owner and also a name!

I phoned up the database to get all the details. It seemed that the dog was actually called Penny, so I hadn't been too far out with my pseudonym of Poppy. I was anxious to speak to the owners as soon as possible. They must surely have been distraught with worry, and I wanted to let them know that although she was badly injured, she was safe and alive. However, worse news was to follow — the only telephone number recorded on the database did not work. It had too few digits. Optimistically, I typed the name into the practice system, but there were no pointers called Penny. After all, I had picked her up quite a long way from Thirsk, so she was unlikely to be a patient of ours. I wondered if I should telephone the veterinary surgeries in that area to ask them to check their records, but by now it was half past eleven at night. I could imagine exactly how unpopular I would be if I woke up at least four on-duty veterinary surgeons and demanded that they go back into work to check their computer systems. I would not be able to trace Penny's owners until morning.

Now, though, I needed to turn my attention to Penny's leg. I had already managed to get an intravenous catheter into the vein in her good leg, through which I was running a saline drip to treat the inevitable shock from which she was suffering. She was quiet and relaxed, still under sedation, so I set about taking some x-rays to see whether the leg was fractured or the shoulder dislocated or both. It is vital to replace a dislocation as soon as possible, otherwise it becomes very hard to do, and much more likely to pop out again. Quick replacement is also the very best form of analgesia, as every rugby player who has experienced a dislocated shoulder will know.

But the x-ray did not show a dislocation. Rather there was, as I had feared, a nasty fracture to the humerus (the long bone between the shoulder and the elbow). The middle part of the bone was completely smashed. This led me to my next dilemma. Stabilising a fracture is always the first priority, as it is the best form of pain relief and stops further tissue damage. The bone clearly needed to be repaired. Fractures can either be repaired immediately, before much of the bruising and swelling has had time to set in, or a day or two later after the swelling has subsided. There are arguments either way as to which is best, but in this case the injury was so high up the leg that I was going to struggle to stabilize it properly in any way other than by just getting on and fixing it. However, as I hadn't managed to find an owner, I couldn't get their consent for surgery. Should I just carry on anyway? There was always a possibility they would not want surgery but prefer to go for amputation or even euthanasia. What to do?

Fixing a fracture is usually a two-man job. I did have a second on-call vet on the other end of the phone, who I knew I should really contact to come in and help. But I also knew he had been on call the previous night and had the weekend ahead to cover. Penny was nicely sedated so it would be fairly easy to administer an anaesthetic injection via the catheter that was already in place. I decided I could press on alone. That way I would save him another disturbed night's sleep.

I thought I could manage singlehandedly, if I was careful with my planning and efficient with my surgery. Once Penny's anaesthetic was stable, I could clip and scrub the leg, open my equipment then scrub my hands and arms and don surgical gloves. I would open up every single bit of equipment I thought I might need — plenty of pre-sterilised packs of plates, screws, pins and orthopaedic wire — so that I wouldn't need a nurse or an assistant to pass them to me. Whilst this would be very much frowned upon by the purists, I reasoned that even under my sole charge, things were still a million times better for Penny than they had been three hours ago.

So I made a decision and made a start.

The anaesthetic was stable and smooth as I made my first incision. The skin was bruised purple by the impact of the lorry and the roughness of the tarmac. The muscle under the skin and around the smashed bone had undergone a colour change that went beyond purple. There were black blood clots all around the smashed-up humerus. I removed the smaller shattered fragments, but carefully retained the bigger pieces so I could fix them back to the intact upper and lower ends of the bone.

My plan was to place an intramedullary pin (a type of metal rod) up the middle of the smashed bone, threading all the pieces back into alignment. It fitted in quite easily and, after about an hour, the two main fragments were more or less together. I used special wire called cerclage wire to keep the other fragments firmly in place. The leg was looking an awful lot better. There was a certain calmness that came over me in the middle of the night, working alone, just Penny and me, the silence only broken by the ticking of the theatre clock and the gentle hiss of the oxygen flowing through the anaesthetic machine. I can recall every moment of that surgery. By the time I had finished, Penny was in an immeasurably better place than she had been at the start of the evening.

After she had woken up from her operation, I plied her with yet more morphine and other painkilling medication and carried her to her new kennel so that she could recover slowly from her operation. Then I headed for home. It was three o'clock in the morning and I had missed my tea, and hadn't seen my kids or my wife. It had been a busy day and a long night and I was exhausted. I fell into bed and was instantly asleep.

Morning came all too quickly. I rushed in to work to check on Penny, before my beeper could go off again and take me in a different direction. In her kennel at the practice she was sitting up and looking around. She seemed like a new dog altogether. I looped a lead over her head for a second time in twelve hours and took her outside for a walk and a wee. This would be the first test of her leg and of my surgery. Penny was hesitant but walked out gingerly, sniffing the air as if trying to work out where on earth she was. I imagine the morphine haze had left her confused and bewildered. The last thing she would have remembered must have been seeing the radiator grille of the lorry on the A1, and now she was here, at my clinic and very sore. Outside in the spring air, I could see her spirits lift. Three of her legs worked well (this was good news, for I had not examined them in great detail the previous night) and the left fore was bruised and battered but taking a little of her weight.

Now it was of utmost importance to trace her owners. I had my morning appointments to do, but by the time I had completed my list of consultations Rachel, the head nurse, had tracked them down and I had a phone call to make.

The best bit about being a veterinary surgeon is seeing the animals feel better. The second best bit is relaying this news to worried owners. It was no different this time. I need not have worried about jumping headlong into serious orthopaedic surgery without the prior consent of

Penny's owner. Elaine was overjoyed that Penny had been found, that I had operated so promptly and that she was now doing well. Penny had escaped from the family garden, she explained, as pointers tend to do, and had evidently run off in search of adventure. The collar that she usually wore bearing her name, address and telephone number must have got lost in a hedge as Penny raced around the fields of North Yorkshire. Elaine was at the practice to see her beloved dog within the hour, just as soon as she had updated her details on the microchip database.

I made another phone call, too, this time to Sheila. She had spent so much time with Penny at the side of the road and was delighted to hear that the story had ended happily.

It wasn't quite the end of the story. The biggest test would be the healing of Penny's leg. Over the next few months I saw a lot of her, removing the sutures from her wound and managing her recovery. I removed the pin under anaesthetic three months after the accident. The bone was straight, firm and pain-free. The power of the body to re-form from a mangled mess never fails to astonish me. As surgeons, we are simply there to offer nature a helping hand.

I still see Penny regularly. It is a joy to see her happy and well and back to normal. Penny, though, seems stubbornly oblivious to my involvement in saving her and her leg, and resolutely refuses to wag her tail in my direction.

I blame it on the morphine.

Ripe Tomatoes

The end of springtime signals the end of lambing time. The young lambs run and jump around in the spring fields, a summer of growing and getting fat ahead of them. But as shepherds breathe a sigh of relief, beef suckler farmers, whose cows have calved in the spring, are beginning to think about the condition of their bull. Once summer arrives the bull will be in action, making sure the cows become pregnant again. Modern, well-managed herds like to have their bulls tested for fertility before putting them back with the cows, so that no time is lost if there is a problem. This is a relatively simple procedure, with the right skills and equipment.

One of our suckler herds had experienced a huge problem the previous year. Out of a batch of about fifty cows, that had spent the summer with a single bull, not one calf was born. The bull was infertile. It was a disaster. The following spring, the farm manager asked if I would fertility test all five Aberdeen Angus bulls, to check they were okay. I didn't have the required tools, and I hadn't done this job before, but a few months previously, at a veterinary conference, I had met a veterinary surgeon called Fraser from a practice over in the Yorkshire Wolds. He had all the kit and all the expertise, and had offered his services should the need ever arise. I found his number and gave him a call.

He was happy to help.

So, on a lovely sunny spring day I found myself waiting on the farm chatting to the farmers, while a collection of onlookers, including someone's ten-year-old son, gathered to watch the spectacle that was the fertility testing of five enormous bulls. It wasn't long before an estate car appeared, driving down the daffodil-lined farm track. In those days, the seniority of a large animal vet could be measured by the size of his estate car and Fraser's did not disappoint.

He pulled up right next to the cattle crush where the first bull was waiting patiently, utterly oblivious to what was in store for him.

Fraser leapt out of the vehicle and, with great gusto, shook hands with everyone.

'What a glorious day for a job like this!' he enthused in a soft Scottish accent.

It was, indeed, a beautiful day. The warm spring sunshine made it a joy to be outside in the fresh air. It was almost possible to see the grass growing. I hoped this spring feeling would make the bulls turn their attention to the task in hand.

As we spoke, a very glamorous lady appeared from the passenger seat of the estate car.

'Oh, I'm terribly sorry. I must introduce my wife. This is Kirsty.'

Kirsty had come along to act as assistant. Successful fertility testing requires the help of someone who knows what to do and Fraser had worked out that neither the farm staff nor I had ever done this kind of thing before. I was hoping to learn a lot today (Fraser had assured me on the phone that, having watched five bulls being tested one after another, I too would soon be an expert), but it was sure to run more smoothly with some experienced help.

Before long everything was set up. There was a table, on which there was a microscope with a heated panel to keep the semen sample at the correct temperature. There was also an incubator so the various other liquids could be kept at the right temperature too, because if at any stage during the testing process the sample was to become too hot, or too cold, the sperm would simply die and give an erroneously negative test. The main bit of equipment though, was the electro-ejaculator. It was a yellow, white and metallic-coloured torpedo-shaped device, about the size of a small marrow. It was amply lubricated and carefully inserted into the bull's rectum. A small electrical current was applied to stimulate the prostate and produce a semen sample. It sounds horrendous, but the modern equipment is actually very gentle and the bulls do not mind the procedure at all.

However, before the extraordinary moment when the electro-ejaculator was brought into action, Fraser palpated the bull's testicles and internal, accessory sex organs. He dictated copious notes to his glamorous assistant, in much the same way as a dentist dictates to the dental nurse while probing your teeth.

'Julian, the testicles need to be the consistency of ripe tomatoes — not too soft, you see?' Fraser explained. I made a mental note: 'ripe tomatoes'.

He then went on to measure the circumference

of the bull's scrotum, all the time explaining what he was doing.

'Whatever you do, don't squeeze them too hard.'

'Okay, must remember not to squeeze them too hard,' I repeated inside my head.

'If you squeeze them too hard, you get a measurement that is too low. Scrotal circumference is strongly correlated with reproductive performance.'

I made another mental note. I was already the father of two sons but until this moment, I had never given scrotal circumference a second thought.

After this part of the assessment, we all got the feeling that the big moment had arrived. First, though, there was another little job to be done. Kirsty opened the side door of the cattle crush, bent down and pulled a pair of shiny, curved scissors from her pocket.

'I always like to give them a quick trim,' she explained as she set about trimming all the extraneous hair from the bull's prepuce.

'There. That's much better.'

She stood up and admired her work, which was, it had to be said, immaculate. The raised eyebrows from the assembled crowd did not have time to resume their normal position, as it was now time for the real action. Fraser carefully inserted the probe and everybody, including ten-year-old Charlie, watched with amazement. As Fraser fiddled with the control panel, providing exactly the correct level of stimulation in a rhythmic fashion, the bull was gently coaxed into action. Kirsty positioned the catching tube. It was conveniently attached to a funnel on the end of a long plastic handle so she could hold it safely under the bull, right in front of his penis, ready to catch the sample. Lo and behold, after a few minutes, the bull ejaculated and Kirsty expertly collected it all in her tube. With much excitement, Fraser switched off the machine and exclaimed: 'Come on, Julian. It's time to look down the microscope!'

I hurried after him.

'There's not a moment to be wasted,' he shouted over his shoulder. 'We need to look at it before it gets too cold.'

Off we scurried towards the little office where the microscope and incubator had been set up. Once we arrived, Fraser quickly dropped little blobs of the sample onto several glass slides. Some had tiny glass cover slips placed carefully over them, while others were mixed with purple dye to be analysed later. That way the shape and structure of each sperm could be checked in detail. The most pressing job, though, was to check for motility and the first sample proved to be superb.

'What a corker! Look at this!'

Fraser beckoned me over to the microscope. I could see swirling, dark grey patterns, moving just like the smoke from a leafy bonfire on a gusty day.

'That', explained Fraser, 'is a four out of five for gross motility. It is very good. This is a great sample. A beauty!'

He explained all about gross motility and

104

progressive motility and the other morphological tests he would need to do later, back at his practice.

We repeated the process with the other four bulls but I was already captivated by the simplicity of the testing and the immediacy of the results. I had always loved the science of cytology — looking at cells down a microscope. To see the basic building blocks of a body is an amazing thing, but to see the cells that could be the beginning of the life of a new calf was utterly breathtaking. I was hooked.

After we had finished the final bull, I thanked Fraser and Kirsty for their time and enthusiasm and for Fraser's tuition. Fraser assured me again that, with some more reading and the right equipment, I would soon be competent at doing the tests myself. I rushed straight back to the practice to search the internet for the required kit and, by the end of the week, I had also enrolled on a course. I would soon be knowledge-able and equipped enough to test all the bulls of Thirsk.

The Perils of Grass

By the middle of April, cattle farmers are thinking about letting their cattle out to graze. The precise timing of this takes good judgement, for whilst there is an impatience to get the animals back to their natural diet of grass and to free them from the confines of the farm buildings, there can be some nasty meteorological stings in the tail of spring, even after April has passed. If the weather turns bad after the cattle are let out, or if the paddocks are too boggy, the consequences can be serious. A field of delicate spring grass can quickly be churned up into a sea of mud, rendering it useless for much of the summer. The timing is critical. One wise old farmer advised me, following the advice given to him by his father, not to consider winter to be over (in this case, 'winter' referring to the time that cattle are housed, rather than simply one of the four seasons) until May had passed! This seemed remarkably pessimistic to me but the philosophy did, at least, ensure that there was always sufficient winter fodder on this farm to keep the cattle well fed, even through the worst and wettest of springs.

Eventually though, coldness and wetness gives way to warmth and cattle are let out of their gloomy sheds and turned out to grass. They rush out with great excitement, bucking and kicking in a very ungainly but completely joyful fashion.

It is just the same when young lambs go outside for the first time. It is an exciting time for a vet too, although we don't usually run and jump as we make our way around our calls. Lighter nights, longer days and warmer hands for the next six months makes spring a joyous time to be a vet in mixed practice.

The change of diet for cows from silage to grass makes its own special type of veterinary excitement.

In some ways the digestive system of a ruminant is extremely robust. The rumen is a large fermentation chamber, full of microbes capable of digesting all sorts of plant material that other animals simply would not be able to digest. It is a symbiotic relationship — the bugs get a free home inside the rumen of this gentle creature and the cow gets its food digested more easily. The number and type of bugs adapt to the type of food that a ruminant is fed, so whilst the system works very well for both cow and microbe, it struggles to cope with a sudden change in diet. Therefore, the most common problem facing a cow after it heads out to the grassy fields is sloppy, green diarrhoea. This is just a mild inconvenience to the cow and is far outweighed by the benefits of this nutritious leafy food. However, for a veterinary surgeon, it makes any job around the back end of a cow a very messy job indeed. The loose, green faeces splatter everywhere and leave indelible greenish-brown stains that have resulted in many shirts being condemned to the rag bag. Whole herd blood testing, where blood samples are taken from the tail vein of every cow (to test for brucellosis or other diseases) should not be undertaken at this time of the year!

Minor inconveniences aside, there are some more significant problems that can arise as cattle and sheep gorge themselves on the glut of new spring grass.

The most serious of these is called staggers. The warmth of the late April sun on the wet ground makes the grass grow very quickly. After a long winter indoors eating straw and silage, a huge field of thick green grass is a delicious prospect for a cow, but while it looks lush it is, in fact, often depleted in magnesium. The cow quickly fills its stomach with copious quantities of grass that has a high water content and very little magnesium. The body holds no reserves of this mineral so the level in the blood can fall very quickly. The result of this hypomagnesaemia is severe — acute collapse, tremors and convulsions shortly followed by death. As veterinary surgeons, we rarely see them at the staggering stage since the progression of the disease is very rapid, but the cow can be saved by very prompt treatment with intravenous and subcutaneous magnesium solution.

In the days when there were cattle in every field around Thirsk, a warm, damp day at the end of April would spell a constant stream of visits to see cows with staggers. The receptionists were well briefed in the urgency of these cases and would come rushing to find the nearest vet, who would stop whatever they were doing and leap straight into the car.

Such calls were always fraught with excitement and tension. 'Hypomag' cases were satisfying to treat, as long as we were quick. The diagnosis was easy and the response to a bottle of diluted magnesium and calcium solution into the jugular vein, followed by another under the skin, would bring a miraculous recovery, but only if we got there in time.

One of the most spectacular responses I ever saw was in a black and white Friesian cow, belonging to a happy dairy farmer called Wilf. We visited Wilf's farm regularly. Several of his cows, although very well cared for, seemed to suffer from one mineral deficiency or another on a fairly frequent basis. On this particular evening the affected cow was stuck in a field near the banks of the River Swale.

Wilf met me as I drove into the farmyard and waved me towards the field. It was always easier to drive right up to the patient if we could, so we had all our tackle to hand.

'Oh! She's not very good!' shouted Wilf, as I wound down the car window. 'She's shaking and trembling. She's in the field over there. You'll have to follow me. I'll go in the tractor.'

'Can we keep her still, Wilf?' I called, worried we would be chasing a staggering beast round a field with a river running through it. 'Have you got a halter? I'll need to inject her into the vein.'

'Oh no! She can't stand up!' laughed Wilf, and off he went to clamber into the tractor, chuckling to himself and shaking his head, 'Oh no, she can't stand up.'

He always laughed, even in the face of

desperation. Like I said, he was a happy farmer.

Wilf's grandson held the gate open as I headed off across the field, following the tractor. The cow was lying on her side near the river and it was very clear that she had no chance of standing up. She was more likely to tremor and shake herself into the river and float away than she was to get to her feet. Nevertheless, I put a halter on, if nothing else to try to keep her head still so I could give her the medicine that she needed so urgently. Wilf wrapped the end of the rope halter around the front of his tractor to keep her fastened.

The cow was very close to death. The treatment was to drip nearly half a litre of magnesium solution very slowly into the jugular vein, using a long orange rubber tube called a flutter valve. The flutter valve connected to the bottle of magnesium at one end and the needle in the vein at the other. It required a steady hand to keep the needle in place, and at the same time to hold the bottle up to the right height. The higher the bottle is held, the faster the magnesium solution runs in, so as well as keeping one hand on the needle and the other on the bottle, it is also crucial to keep one eye on the cow and the other on the rate at which the bottle is emptying. If the solution is run in too quickly, which is easy to do under the pressure of the situation, the medicine that can save the cow's life will stop its heart and cause a fatal heart attack. Too slow, and the effects of insufficient magnesium will kill her. The stakes are high.

So, as the sun was setting and the evening chill taking over from the relative warmth of the afternoon, I watched the elixir glugging in at what I hoped was just the correct rate. The cow stopped shaking and raised herself from lying flat on her side so that she was sitting up. Moments later, and before I had chance to complete the infusion, she rose like Lazarus and charged off, still with the halter fastened snugly around her nose and ears (not so securely fastened to the tractor after all), leaving me with my arm raised above my head, a dangling flutter valve hanging from the bottle in my hand.

'Heavens above, she can't half stand up now!' Wilf guffawed as he burst out laughing. 'She can run as well!'

He was almost rolling around with laughter in the grass, an enormous grin all over his face.

'I'll have to get your halter tomorrow when she comes in for milking! We'll never catch her now!'

And off he went, shaking his head with amusement as he clambered back into the tractor. 'We'll never catch her now!' he continued to chuckle to himself as he started the engine.

★   ★   ★

Another condition that affects milking cows and often goes hand in hand with staggers is called milk fever. Whilst it sounds to the untrained ear like a serious case of lactose intolerance, it is actually caused by a deficiency in calcium. The signs can be similar to staggers and, to

111

complicate matters, both magnesium and calcium deficiency can occur together. However, milk fever is less acute, the treatment is not quite so urgent and the response is not quite as dramatic as it was in Wilf's cow. The low calcium is a result of the large and sudden demand for the mineral in the cow's body, soon after she delivers her calf and starts to produce copious amounts of milk. The result is a muscular weakness that makes the cow unable to stand. It can be serious, because a cow that stays lying on the ground quickly develops all sorts of secondary problems and the outlook deteriorates over just a day or so.

A cow weighing over half a tonne, which cannot stand, can become a logistical nightmare. This was more than evident when I was called early on a Saturday morning to a farm on the far side of Hawnby, a charming but remote little village in the middle of the Hambleton Hills. The cows had been let out for the first night of the year and one, whose name was Buttercup the Third, had not come back in at milking time. The cows would usually stand side by side in the byre to be milked, each one in its correct place, so it was pretty obvious if one of them wasn't there. Brian, the farmer, had set off on his quad bike to find the missing bovine. The field in which the cows had started their grazing season was on a steep slope dotted with gorse bushes.

After much exploration of the hillside, Brian had found Buttercup the Third lying at the bottom of the bank, surrounded by trees and half submerged in an icy stream.

She must have succumbed to the weakening effect of milk fever whilst lying near to the top of the bank and then, as she struggled to rise when the rest of the herd ambled in to be milked, her weak and wobbly legs must have failed her and she had rolled all the way down to the bottom. One could only try to picture the scene of a large and ungainly cow, legs and udder flailing in all directions, somersaulting down the slope, colliding with the occasional gorse bush. Had this happened in the evening as the local pub had shut its doors, the village drinkers would surely have stopped and rubbed their eyes several times to make sure it wasn't a drunken apparition!

But, regardless of how many rolls it had taken and who had seen her on her way down, Buttercup the Third was in a pickle. Breaking every health and safety rule that existed, I perched on the back of Brian's quad bike to reach the stricken cow. I carried all the essential bits of equipment in a plastic bucket. I had the things I would need to make a basic examination and the things I thought I would need to treat the most likely causes of her problem. I took my trusty stethoscope to listen to the heart, lungs and rumen, a thermometer and rectal glove so I could feel inside her abdomen. I also took a flutter valve, bottles of calcium and some needles. I shoved some syringes and other bottles of medicine into my various pockets. I did not want to have to make a second journey up and down the bank.

The diagnosis was fairly straightforward — the swan neck, weak rumen contractions and subnormal temperature were all classic signs of milk fever, although I suspected that, having been sitting in a stream all night, she would have had a low temperature whatever the original cause. I connected up the bottle of calcium to the flutter valve as Brian held her head. She was weak and there was no need for a halter to keep her still. This was lucky, as I'd forgotten to put one in my bucket anyway, so there was no other option than for Brian to cling on to her neck for dear life. The first bottle ran in smoothly and quickly (the mixture of calcium and magnesium together had very little risk of stopping the heart in the way pure magnesium would have done), followed by a second and then a third. In most cases three bottles would be enough to get a cow suffering from milk fever up onto her feet and wandering off to find her friends. But Buttercup the Third showed no signs of moving. There is a sensible limit to how many bottles of calcium it is safe to give a cow over a short period, so I decided to leave it at three and come back to see her again later on that day. Given that some of Buttercup's symptoms were bound to be due to hypothermia brought on by having been in the water for so long, I couldn't be certain exactly how low her calcium levels actually were. It would be risky to give her too much on the first visit.

I told Brian that I would be back, after Saturday morning surgery had finished.

He looked gloomy, mainly because his cow was still lying in a river, but also because he had tickets to watch Middlesbrough play at home that afternoon. I tried to be optimistic about the chances for Buttercup and for Brian's chances of making it to the Riverside for three o'clock, but by the time I had completed morning surgery and negotiated the winding lanes up to Hawnby for the second time, Brian still looked almost as dejected as his cow.

'She's not up, Julian. She's still in the water. She's not even tried to stand.'

Brian's downbeat assessment was quite a contrast to the positive and cheerful attitude of Wilf when his cow was in a similar position, but both Brian and I knew it was a bad sign. A cow that rose to her feet promptly after the medication would always carry a very good prognosis, but the longer she was down, the worse the outlook. The fact that she was lying in a stream and at the bottom of a steep bank made her chances of recovery even more remote. We both knew she might never stand again.

I tried to be positive.

'Not to worry, Brian, I'll give her another three bottles straight into her vein' (that made six in total, so far) ' . . . and some extra phosphorus too. She'll be fine whilst you go to the footie this afternoon. If she needs more, give me a ring and I can come back later this evening.'

'Right you are, Julian,' he replied glumly.

We loaded up the required bottles and I found somewhere to perch on the quad bike for another death-defying ride through the gorse bushes and down the bank. Buttercup the Third was in the same place as before, half in the stream and still lying down. She did look a bit brighter and her large, brown eyes seemed to widen as she saw me clamber off the quad with my bucket of clanking bottles and orange rubber tubing. It was unclear whether this was with excitement of a possible cure or the fear of me sticking my large needle into her neck again.

Half an hour later I'd emptied three more bottles of sticky calcium solution into her jugular vein, followed by twenty millilitres of phosphorus and a syringe of steroids to try and help the bruising she must have suffered as she rolled down the bank. She was sitting on her brisket, but had made no attempts to stand. It was almost as if she was relaxing in the stream and didn't even want to move. Comfortable as she seemed, though, her refusal to rise was worrying and Brian's trip to the Riverside was a very distant prospect.

'Well, you've done all you can, Julian. You've done your best. It's down to her now.'

We clambered back onto the quad bike for the trip back up to the farm.

Poor Buttercup and poor Brian. I felt awful that my medicines hadn't achieved what I had wanted, but offered some reassurance that it might take a while for their full effects to develop.

My beeper intervened at this point. It was a message about a lame cat that needed my attention at the surgery. I had to go. Before I went, I implored Brian to go to the game, to take his mind off Buttercup.

'Give me a ring later tonight and I can come and give her some more calcium,' I offered.

I told him how I had once given a downer cow

116

(that is, one that can't get up) eighteen bottles of calcium before she eventually rose to her feet. The farmer, on that occasion, was utterly unconvinced that it was worth trying so many visits and so many bottles. I had to promise that all the visits would be free if I was unsuccessful. In this case, though, Brian wasn't bothered how many visits it took, just as long as his cow got better. As I left the farm, I knew he would be missing the football match that afternoon. Even if he were to go he wouldn't enjoy it, in the knowledge that the fate of his cow hung in the balance.

Half an hour later, back at the practice, I was treating the lame cat. It had an abscess on its leg as a result of a bite from another cat — a frequent occurrence in springtime when cats stay out late into the evening and get into trouble.

Even though it was painful, it was easy to fix with injections and tablets and I knew this feline patient would be feeling better very quickly, as soon as the medication started to work.

I was frustrated that I hadn't resolved Buttercup's problems just as quickly and easily. I felt as if I had let down Brian and his cow, but the rest of my afternoon was busy and my beeper was rarely quiet, so I didn't have much time to dwell on the recumbent cow and the inadequacies of my treatment.

I didn't hear from Brian again until the middle of Sunday morning.

'Julian, I wonder if you could just come up and have another look at Buttercup, please? If you're not too busy, that is.'

Things had calmed down and, after I had finished attending to the inpatients at the practice, I set off, my car boot replenished with many more brown bottles of calcium solution.

On a lovely sunny morning, the drive to Hawnby is wonderful. The road twists and turns and halfway along there is an enormous hill up onto the moors called Sneck Yate. The drive itself was so pleasant that it hardly seemed like work, as deer hopped out of the woods and across the road in front of the car and horse riders kindly waved me past. I couldn't enjoy the journey as much as I usually did though, as I was certain I would have to euthanase the hopeless case that I would see when I got to the bottom of the wooded bank for the third time in twenty-four hours.

However, to my surprise, when I arrived at the farm Brian's face wore a happier expression. Instead of showing me to the quad bike for the off-road journey I had been expecting, he ushered me through the low-ceilinged cow byre and into the fold yard. It was full of straw and there, sitting comfortably in the middle, chewing on a mouthful of silage, was Buttercup the Third, happy and content.

'I thought you might like to see your old friend,' said Brian, with a wry smile.

'Blimey! How did she get home?'

I was amazed. Surely she hadn't walked all the way up the same steep, gorse-covered bank down which she had rolled over a day ago?

'Well, Julian, after you'd gone, I thought about what I could do to help. I knew she had no chance if I couldn't get her home, so I gave my brother-in-law a ring. He came to give me a hand and we went down the road to the little bridge — the one on the way to Helmsley. We got the chainsaw and took down the hedge so I could get my tractor in. We cut down some holes in the next two hedges and I managed to get my tractor nearly up beside her. We pulled her out and I scooped her up in the bucket.' By this, Brian meant the big metal scoop on the front of the tractor. 'We took her out onto the road and then brought her over the bridge, up the hill and all the way home,' he explained.

For the second time, I could only imagine the expressions on the faces of any villagers who had been sitting in the garden of the pub as a cow came along the road sitting in the front loader of a tractor!

But she was safely returned and had been deposited in a clean, comfy, flat and dry straw yard and she was immeasurably better. She had even been standing up earlier that morning, reported Brian.

'I don't think she needs any more medicine,' he said. 'I just thought you'd like to see her. See what you think.'

Needless to say, Brian had missed the match and had spent his afternoon cutting holes in hedges big enough to fit his tractor through, then repairing the holes again with fencing so the rest of the cows wouldn't escape.

I patted Buttercup on the head and injected her with another dose of phosphorus, before preparing another syringe-full for Brian to inject the next day. We both knew she was, quite literally, out of the woods.

'How was the cat, by the way, Julian?' asked Brian as I climbed back into the car.

'Pretty bad actually, Brian, but I managed to fix her. She only needed two injections!'

Fire Brigade Work

Attending farm animal emergencies, like a cow with staggers or a lambing sheep, is often, in veterinary parlance, referred to as 'fire brigade work'. Some in the veterinary world see this as old-fashioned and the modern protagonists of the profession regard 'herd health' as the way forwards. Veterinary surgeons wielding laptops rather than stethoscopes should have advisory meetings with farmers to discuss nutrition and vaccination, so emergencies do not occur.

In theory this is a great idea, but for small farms like those belonging to Wilf or Brian, providing differential feeding strategies for cows at different stages of their lactation is completely unfeasible. Most of our farmers already use pneumonia vaccination regimes to good effect, so my early forays into the world of 'herd health planning' largely fell on deaf ears. Most of my clients were not convinced and traditional fire brigade work still remains a big part of our daily work.

One visit, not long after I had become a partner at Skeldale, turned out to be more of a 'fire brigade' job than expected.

Harward and David were elderly brothers who ran a small dairy herd on a farm called Village Farm, just outside Thirsk on the way to York. They were both short men and were from the generation of farmers who were always immaculately dressed, wearing a jacket and tie underneath the perennial flat cap. Or rather, Harward's outfits were always topped by a flat cap, as he was the brother who oversaw the outside work. His brother David was in charge of domestic duties — cleaning, washing, cooking, making cups of tea and organizing the paperwork for the farm. It was a curious arrangement.

Our work here was the typical stuff of a small dairy herd: TB testing, cases of mastitis, milk fevers and the odd calving. But the most regular job of all, as it was on many farms like this, was to visit every three weeks to disbud a handful of calves. Calves grow small rubbery buds that will develop into large horns by the time the animal reaches adulthood. Horns are a nuisance because they can easily get knocked and damaged when cows are feeding or going into the milking parlour. More importantly, a cow with horns uses them to bully the other cows, by prodding them in the side. This can cause all sorts of injuries, so it is good practice to remove them when the animals are little calves of about six weeks old, when the job is simpler and less traumatic.

It is a simple enough job. Local anaesthetic is injected into a groove near the horn, where it numbs the nerve that supplies the horn and the top of the head. It takes about ten minutes to take effect and lasts for a few hours, so each calf is numbed first, then we go back round and burn off the horn buds, one calf at a time.

The burning is done using a gas-powered metal burner, with heat coming out of the end, a bit like old-fashioned curling tongs, although with bigger flames. The burner is lit soon after arrival at the farm, so it gets a chance to heat up to the right temperature — it doesn't work very well if it isn't hot enough.

On this particular day, Sue, one of the best vets that I have ever worked with, had put her initials next to the visit to disbud calves at Village Farm and she was there with characteristic promptness and enthusiasm. The brothers liked Sue. She was a whirling dervish of energy and could always put a spring in the step of an elderly farmer. The fact that she could not involve herself with their favourite topic of discussion — cricket — was only a minor inconvenience, and Sue was always welcome. They were happy to miss out on this discussion when Sue burst onto their farm.

Everything was normal at the beginning and the burner was lit up after the usual search for matches. To avoid it being kicked over by the calves, Sue had positioned the burner in the next pen, where it was also out of the draught coming down the passage. Each one of the calves was injected and the conversation was in full flow.

Suddenly the mood changed, as smoke appeared from the neighbouring pen and it became evident that something was on fire. It was in the days before mobile phones, so David rushed into the house to call the fire brigade and immediately Sue and Harward stopped what they were doing to tackle the fire.

The burner had set fire to the straw and the wooden feed trough was alight, too. With luck, Sue managed to grab the burner and pull it out of the blaze, turn it off and sling it into the grass outside the Dutch barn. Harward, normally cool and calm under the pressure of a sick cow or a difficult calving, panicked and ran off in the opposite direction, presumably looking for water.

By the time he returned with a half-full bucket, the flames were near the wooden roof struts and disaster was close at hand. Half a bucket of water didn't achieve very much and Harward ran off again to get more, shouting at the top of his voice.

Luckily, on this particular morning the fire brigade in Thirsk was not very busy. Sirens were heard, and blue lights soon appeared outside the farm. The firemen unravelled their hosepipes just as flames were lapping the top of the calf pen. Disaster had been averted.

After cups of tea all round, two of them fortified with brandy, the firemen were on their way and the rest of the job was completed.

Back at the practice, there was some concern. The senior partner was blustering around.

'Where's Sue got to? She's been gone all morning and she only had half a dozen calves to disbud! She needs to get back here and finish off the ops list! What's taking her so long?'

Little did we know what had happened until Sue reappeared, tousled and smoky. She related the story, finishing by saying pitifully, 'Julian, I was absolutely gutted.'

I expected her to explain how mortified she had been to inflict such devastation on a small farm and how close to disaster it had been, but no.

'I was out on call early this morning and I then found myself surrounded by all these lovely firemen and I hadn't even had chance to put my make-up on!'

Luna the Easter Bunny

I'd spent much of Easter Sunday out on visits. Easter weekend is always busy with lambings and calvings and the inevitable accidents and injuries that ensue as people get out and about in the spring sunshine on their horses, or with their dogs. When I eventually returned home, I caught the tail end of a family argument. Archie, my youngest son, who was ten, came stomping down the stairs clutching his moneybox and looking grumpy. Jack, his older brother, had struck a deal with him to pay half of an annual membership to Xbox Live, and was shouting at him from the sitting room.

'Archie, you owe Mum twenty pounds. She's paid it on her credit card.'

My wife Anne was puzzled. She couldn't work out why Archie was upset. I put the kettle on and listened, trying to keep out of it. I kept well clear of all things to do with both computer games and their online subscriptions. It was not my department. I could imagine Jack's canny trick though, because I remembered brokering a similar deal with my younger sister, Kate, many years ago when I was about the same age. I had persuaded her to buy a large supply of my spare 'swaps' of *Star Wars* cards. Poor Kate had no interest in *Star Wars* whatsoever, but such is the persuasive power of an older brother.

'What's the matter, Archie?' asked Anne. 'I

thought you had agreed this with Jack?'

Tears welled up in Archie's eyes.

'I don't want Xbox Live. None of my friends play on it, and all those games Jack plays are twelve certificates and I'm not allowed to play on them . . . and anyway . . . '

Then came the killer blow.

' . . . I'm saving up for a rabbit!'

He had his mother right where he wanted her. He had just said he had no interest in the computer and wanted a fluffy pet instead. What parent could object to such a beautifully clear argument? Archie was a genius. So either by design, cunning or good fortune the die was cast. He started researching rabbits. How to care for them, what to feed them, what to do, what not to do, and the next thing I knew, I arrived home for lunch one day the following week to find a luxury hutch being assembled in the kitchen.

Archie had saved up enough money and a date was set for the purchase of the fluffy pet. I wasn't that keen on rabbits. My main experiences of them were as nervous, stricken pets often having been confined to a tiny little hutch at the end of a garden, long since forgotten about by a child who had grown up and moved on to other things. I did not want this fate to befall a rabbit under our care.

'Have we discussed getting this rabbit?' I ventured to Anne when Archie, by now in full rabbit mode, was out of earshot. Usually these things necessitated a lengthy family debate. At least as much debate as the acquisition of the blooming Xbox. I didn't want that either.

'Well, I told you he was saving up for one. He's already got the guinea pigs so it won't make that much difference. You can't tell him he can't have one now!'

So before the Easter holidays came to an end, off they went to choose the rabbit. I was at work (as usual). We had decided in advance that it should be male, and that we (I) would castrate it. Female rabbits can be bad-tempered, and spaying them is a risky business. Halfway through the morning, my phone rang. It was Anne.

'Well, he's found one he likes, but it's female — what shall I do?'

I pondered for a moment or two, before giving my well-considered veterinary answer.

'Is it cute?'

'Well, it's definitely the best one — it came straight up to him, and seems fit and healthy.'

I spoke to Archie.

'Arch, can you send me a photo?'

A moment or two later, my phone pinged, and a picture of a little white rabbit with brown spots and big ears appeared on the screen, standing up on her back legs and peering at the camera.

'Cute enough,' I texted back. 'Get that one.'

And so Luna arrived to join the two guinea pigs and the dog. It was the start of a wonderful friendship. Between me and a rabbit.

To say Luna was cute was an absolute understatement. Tiny and fluffy and endearing, we all fell in love with her as soon as she arrived. Archie immediately spruced up her hutch. It was large and cosy in equal measure and nestled in a sheltered spot in the garden. Her next present was an outdoor run so she could play on the grass and eat its healthy lush stems. The correct feeding of rabbits is critical to their health. The natural diet of a rabbit is based almost entirely on grass and any significant deviation from this main foodstuff can lead to severe deficiencies and ill health. There was some pioneering research undertaken by Francis Harcourt-Brown, a veterinary surgeon from Harrogate who specialized in rabbits, in the 1990s. She showed that wild rabbits — which ate exclusively grass — had skulls with the correct amount of bone strength. Pet rabbits fed on the muesli-type diet beloved of many pet shops at the time developed weak bones both in their skull and the rest of their skeleton, making them prone to spinal fractures and, just as bad, loose teeth. This was also shown to be a key risk factor in the development of dental and facial abscesses, as bacteria could invade the delicate structures and cause havoc.

Luna, we resolved, would have a diet full of large amounts of grass through most of the year. Good quality feeding hay would support her nutritional needs in the winter when there wasn't much grass, and pelleted rabbit food — just an eggcupful a day, Archie assured me — should then be all she would need, with extra treats comprising dandelions, parsley, mint, basil, rocket and anything else left over from the vegetable patch. Oh, and the odd branch from an apple or pear tree so she could nibble on the bark. Luna was all set to be the healthiest rabbit on the planet.

We put the outdoor pen on the lawn, right up

close to the one that the guinea pigs — Sparkle and Shine — lived in during the day. Their outdoor pen was shaped like a Toblerone, with an outside and an inside compartment, and they would scurry and squeak in and out, taking sneaky peeks at their new friend, just the same size as them, but fluffier and with bigger ears. They had never seen a rabbit before, but it was clear by watching their curious and inquisitive behaviour that they approved of the new addition. They could just about get their noses together through the wire. Despite all Archie's information stating that rabbits and guinea pigs should NEVER be mixed, we couldn't really see why it would be a problem. The pigs were pretty robust and Luna was only little. Under close supervision, the three of them were soon happily eating grass together in Luna's larger outdoor pen. The guinea pig Toblerone hutch was looking for a new home — it was too small for the three of them.

A few weeks later I went to do a house visit to see Blackie, a stray cat that had been adopted by one of our neighbours. He was still quite nervous and timid, so was living in an outbuilding. Blackie needed a health check, some blood tests, his vaccinations and some worming treatment, so I had taken him back to the practice in a cat basket, and returned with him later that day. His owner was delighted and we spent quarter of an hour or so in the garden, as Blackie rushed back to the safety of his shed. I couldn't help but notice, at the bottom of their garden, a rather splendid wire enclosure, which housed about five pet ducks. It was almost big enough for an adult to stand up in, it had a detachable plastic roof and a door which could be opened and closed from both inside and out. It looked just the thing for two guinea pigs and a little white rabbit. I got the details, and before the end of the week, the third rabbit house had arrived in a massive flat pack. We had spent more money on the half-kilogram ball of fluff in just two weeks than we had ever invested in any other family pet!

Once it had been expertly built by Jack, the animals had a magnificent place to play. It was big enough for an array of toys — tubes to hide in, balls to push around and platforms of different levels on which Luna could climb. I would often go in, sit on an upturned bucket with my cup of tea and talk to her. She was more interested in my conversation than Sparkle and Shine were — they mostly just liked eating. We covered all the main topics of conversation during that first springtime, over a lunchtime sandwich or occasionally a post-work gin and tonic (both of those for me, not the rabbit). Luna knew all the clinical conundrums that I had come across during the day and she wrinkled up her nose and licked my hand as if to offer support.

As Luna grew older and bigger, Anne, Archie and I knew she needed to be spayed. Anne, although a very competent veterinary surgeon herself, completely refused to undertake the operation, not being keen on operating on her own pets. The job would clearly fall to me and it was not one that I was looking forward to.

Rabbits are traditionally viewed as having an increased anaesthetic risk compared with other animals. Statistically, the risk of an anaesthetic death in a healthy dog is about one in two thousand. Rabbits don't compare well, with their chances of not waking up from surgery as high as about one in eighty. So, putting a rabbit under anaesthetic is not something to enter into lightly — especially when it is the favourite pet of your youngest son and also your new tea-drinking companion.

We had explained the pros and cons to Archie in great detail. A female rabbit is very much more healthy if she is spayed. The risk of uterine and ovarian cancer is eliminated by having a rabbit spayed since those organs are completely removed. Given that this type of cancer is the commonest cause of life-limiting illness in female rabbits, that alone is a justifiable reason. Rabbits that are not spayed come into season and become bad-tempered and unpleasant companions for guinea pigs and grumpy pets for their owners. In short, we all knew the operation was important, but it didn't make the day of Luna's visit to the clinic any easier.

Manfully, Archie brought Luna into the practice on his way to school. He openly admitted that he wouldn't be able to concentrate on his lessons all day.

'Take your phone, Arch,' I suggested. 'I'll give you a ring at playtime to let you know how she is.'

Taking mobile phones into school wasn't really allowed, but I thought we could swerve the strict rules today. Archie took a deep breath as he stroked Luna's fluffy head and said goodbye.

'I know she's in good hands,' he said bravely as he got back into the car to go to school.

Twenty minutes later, I took an equally deep breath and made my first incision. The scalpel did its work with typical precision and I was soon peering inside the abdomen of my fluffy little friend, probing carefully with forceps to identify her uterus. Luna was a healthy, young rabbit. She had an impeccable diet, ran around a lot and got plenty of fresh air. There was not a trace of the excessive abdominal fat that we often find, which can make surgery like this more complicated. I glanced up at India, our new trainee nurse, for reassurance about the anaesthetic. A nod put me at ease. I tried not to alert India to the fact that I was more anxious than usual, although due to the uncharacteristic tremor of my hands, she knew full well that I would only be happy when this patient was sitting up again, munching on her pile of basil and mint.

The surgery went perfectly and, despite my nerves, Luna was indeed soon back in recovery, her head lolling on top of the optimistically placed pile of herbs that Archie had carefully collected before school. It is important that rabbits start eating quite soon after they wake up from an anaesthetic, so the intestines continue to work, but at this stage the foliage was more useful as a pillow for her weary head.

My phone was back in action as I 'WhatsApp-ed' a picture of our favourite rabbit to Archie.

'She's fine, Arch. Everything's gone well. Have

a good day at school,' I typed at the bottom of the photo.

'Thanks, Dad,' came the immediate and phlegmatic reply that could only come from a ten-year-old boy. 'I'm glad she's not dead.'

The Last Lamb of Spring

'And you'd better be bloody quick abart it, too!' were the last few words I heard before the telephone went dead.

This was ironic because Dave North had just spent the last twenty-five minutes talking me through the problems that this particular sheep was having, as well as the lambing problems of the last half a dozen sheep on his farm. He was renowned within the practice for his lengthy telephone conversations and this morning's chat was no different. Had he been as succinct as most farmers were when they had a ewe to lamb, I would already have been kneeling beside the sheep and the lambs would probably already have been delivered.

So as soon as I'd finished my lengthy conversation, I wrote the visit in the daybook, signed my initials next to it and before long I was in my car, heading out to see him and his sheep. I was already steeling myself for a barrage of thoughts and theories about every imaginable farming and animal-related topic. Dave had a lot of theories.

Once I arrived at the end of his farm track, it took a further full ten minutes before I pulled up outside the farmhouse — an impressive stone and brick building that looked as if it dated back to the seventeenth century — because the track was one of those that wound through fields and

135

therefore had a multitude of gates. These tracks are the nemesis of a vet in a hurry. Stop, climb out of car, open gate, climb back into car, drive through, stop, climb out of car, close gate, climb into car, drive fifty metres and repeat — as many times as there are gates. My first experience of gated farm tracks like this was when I was a veterinary student seeing practice in Skipton. The senior partner was heading out to calve a heifer and he went out of his way to come and find me.

'Ah! You must be the student.'

Although I hadn't been keeping a low profile, I had not spent any time with the senior vet, who was called Ian. He always seemed to be busy and I didn't want to get in his way and slow him up.

'Would you like to come and see this calving with me? It's a bit of a trek, but this farmer is good at calving his cows, so if he's called us in, it's likely to be a caesarian. You should come along.'

I was pleased to have been asked, so I wasted no time in leaping into his four-by-four, even though it was a cold and dark March evening, just before the surgery was about to shut up for the night. I should have been getting on my bike to cycle back to the caravan that was acting as my lodgings for the fortnight.

The farm was right on the top of a moor and it was a cold and windy night. My job, it turned out, was not to fill syringes or assist with the surgery, but to open about twenty gates that were dotted every few hundred metres across the moor. By about the fifth I had worked this out.

'I see why you wanted me to come to experience this calving now!' I said and the serious face of the older vet cracked into a smile.

'Yes, you're right! But it's a great help to me — you've saved me loads of time.'

The lane to Dave's farm wasn't quite as long as that one had been, but its gates were, nonetheless, numerous and it took me some time to reach the farm, where I expected to find Dave marching backwards and forwards impatiently, outside his lambing shed. But there was nobody around at all, so I went to knock on the door of the impressive farmhouse.

'Come in,' was the unusually terse response from within the kitchen. I ventured inside.

'Ah! You're here,' he continued, looking relieved. 'Thanks for coming. She's having a few problems and I'll be bloody buggered if I can lamb her. Too much of a bloody job for me, I'm afraid.'

Dave looked just like Claude Greengrass from the television programme *Heartbeat*. He was rather rotund, with bushy hair and, as he stood up from the kitchen table at which he had been sitting, it became evident he was wearing a long coat fastened around his middle with bailer twine. His cigar stayed in his mouth through all of this introductory chat.

'She's in here,' he explained and I expected him to don his wellies and show me to the nearby farm building. But Dave walked from the kitchen into the adjacent utility room, in which there was a washing machine, a medicine cabinet and a lambing pen made of wooden hurdles along two sides, the other two sides being the washing machine and the wall.

'It's cold out and I thought she stood a better bloody chance in here where it was warm,' he said, sensing that I was surprised to see a sheep in the house.

'Okay. Well, let's have a look. Has she been on long?'

'Oh, she started last night. That's when I brought her in. I've been watching her all night and nowt's happened. That's why you're here. She's abart bloody buggered, poor lass. That's why I wanted you as soon as possible.'

The poor ewe did look exhausted from her attempts to give birth, lying as she was in the straw-lined pen, between the kitchen appliances. At least there was a hot tap nearby and I wasted no time in filling up my bucket with warm water for a change. This was shaping up to be a luxurious lambing experience and one that I would never forget!

After cleaning my hands and applying lubricant, I felt for the lamb. It was very clear why the sheep was not managing on her own. The lamb was enormous.

'Dave, this lamb is massive. It's never going to come out this way. We'll need to do a caesarian.'

Well, it was as if I had just suggested that Dave sold his mother into slavery. He had very little knowledge or experience of this operation, and the idea obviously filled him with fear.

'Oh, I'm not so sure abart that! Can you not get it art t' normal route?'

'Dave, the lamb is massive and that is why it's

not coming. Everything is lined up. The head and front legs are there, but it's just too big. I can pull and pull with my lambing ropes, but it'll never come out this way. Honest.'

Dave pulled heavily on his cigar, which seemed incongruous both because he was standing beside a washing machine and because it was still early in the day. It did, however, give him pause for thought.

'Well, okay. It needs to bloody well come art and if that's the only bloody way, it's the only way. What do we do now?'

'It's fine, I'll need some more warm water and I'll get my stuff — don't worry, it's pretty straightforward.'

I gathered all my tackle — local anaesthetic, surgical kit, various injections and the all-important suture materials — and arranged the ewe so that she was lying on her right side with her left hind leg hoisted upwards, exposing her lower abdomen and groin. I explained to Dave, briefly, what I would be doing. If everything went according to plan, I would be finished in less than fifteen minutes.

I loaded the scalpel onto its handle and prepared for my first incision. At this point, bizarrely, the recollection of the first caesarian section I ever experienced came to mind, maybe because this was the first time Dave had seen the procedure, too.

I was a fifteen-year-old schoolboy and was just coming to the end of a two-day placement at a local veterinary surgery in Wakefield. A yellow Labrador retriever was giving birth and the pups were not coming out as they should. The vet in charge, a brilliant surgeon called Peter Rhodes, was supervising. I should have left the practice an hour or so previously, to catch my bus home, but the prospect of watching this amazing operation was too exciting.

The bitch was placed under anaesthetic and her belly clipped and scrubbed. After just a few moments, Peter was making the same cut that I was about to make into the animal's abdomen to reveal the distended uterus, full of puppies. I was enthralled by the spectacle and was peering in, as close as I dared. Just moments after Peter had made his incision, the bitch did a series of big puffs on the anaesthetic gas. This made the diaphragm contract and the result was that the mass of small intestines spewed out of the abdomen and headed straight towards my face! Clearly the intestines were well and truly attached to the inside of the Labrador and there was no danger of them spilling further than the draped area on the operating table, but I was a naïve schoolboy. Instinct took over and, oblivious to the sterility within the operating site, I stuck out my hands and caught the dog's intestines. My games teacher at school would have been proud, but Mr Rhodes was not. In fact, he was furious. Prone to occasional bad language, even within the consulting room with clients, Peter let out a great torrent of expletives, not aimed directly at me, but at the general situation. As he summoned bags of sterile solution to wash any germs from the dog's insides, I quickly realized my mistake and my face flushed a deep shade of crimson. It was a lesson well learnt.

If intestines spilled out today, I did not want Dave and his cigar reaching out to catch them. Luckily for the sheep and for me, we were on the floor of the utility room and Dave was perched against the washing machine. I knew full well that he was not quick or agile enough to dive to the rescue.

Dave talked continuously throughout the surgery, so much so that his cigar lost its light. I was concentrating hard on what I was doing, so there was precious little opportunity to reply or interject as he extolled his thoughts and theories about all aspects of life.

The operation went smoothly, and one enormous lamb was soon spluttering in the straw next to the washing machine, shaking its head and splattering the kitchen units with bloody mucus.

Dave didn't seem to have any intention of moving the mother and baby out of the house and back to the proper place for a sheep and lamb, and he continued talking. I gathered up my kit and went out to find the hosepipe to clean off. I knew I would be on the farm for some time yet.

'And I'll tell you another bloody thing, that bullock you saw last year, you know, the one with the lump on its side, well, that bloody lump on that bloody bullock, it never did go away. And do you know what I think it was? I think it was — now I might be wrong here, but I don't think I am — I think that lump was a big bloody version of a . . . '

Dave paused and I dared not imagine what his next conjecture might be. I considered running away to my car, but that seemed rude.

He took a deep draw on his long-dead cigar before uttering the unlikely words: 'Lumpy jaw. I think it was a bloody version of lumpy jaw. I do.'

'Well, it might have been, Dave. Where was the lump again?' I could not bring to mind the particular lump to which he was referring.

'That bloody lump was right on the end of his shoulder.'

It seemed unlikely that a lump on the shoulder was a version of the distinctly different condition called 'lumpy jaw', a chronic bacterial infection of the mandible, but Dave was convinced and I knew Dave well enough to know that to disagree was futile. I also knew that it would be a while before I was retracing my steps down his long farm track. When I did eventually manage to get away, I couldn't help but smile at the outcome of my caesarian in the utility room, Dave's cheerfully persistent conviction that he had the answers and the beautiful hawthorn blossom on the hedge along his lane. I knew that once this final lambing of the year had been done, at Dave's farm, springtime was officially over.

Summer

The first thing we all do when we arrive at the practice in the morning is check the daybook, to see what the day has in store. All the operations are listed first, sometimes going over onto a second page. After these come messages and appointments, followed by a list of visits. In a practice like ours, every day is different.

On a sunny summer's day, we all secretly long to get our initials next to a 'plum' job such as forty or fifty sheep to blood sample, outside in the fresh air, with an opportunity to soak up the sun. Apart from performing fifty squats — bending down and standing up each time a sample is taken — a job like this is not physically demanding. There is zero risk of getting debilitating cold fingers or freezing feet, and every chance of getting a suntan.

Bingo and Bertie

It was shaping up to be a beautiful day, and I scoured the pages of the daybook, searching for an outside call. But I was out of luck. Sue had already put her name next to the visit to disbud a gang of young calves and Ben, whose main interest was in equines, was, as ever, heading off to one of the yards to vaccinate some horses and contemplate the cause of lameness in a Shetland pony, before prescribing his usual treatment.

'Nice trousers,' Sue commented as she glanced back over her shoulder on her way out. 'Very summery.'

My trousers were indeed quite summery, although not intentionally so. Once upon a time they were the standard beige corduroy that is practically the uniform for a rural vet. Along with a checked shirt, the outfit is a classic and for good reason. Trousers of any brown shade hide the suspicious stains that would send trousers of any other colour straight to the laundry basket. Similarly, a shirt with numerous lines, vertical and horizontal, can easily fool the eye into an appearance of relative cleanliness. The combination is popular for vets who spend much of their time out on farms.

Today, though, was the first outing of the trousers sporting their new lighter colour. It was around the time when our first son was a baby and the washing basket was permanently full.

The sorting of the washing hadn't gone quite according to plan and a bright blue baby outfit had sneaked in with my favourite and most comfortable pair of trousers. When they emerged from the washing machine, they had changed from a modest brown to a bright turquoise, rendering them utterly useless for wearing in public. Anne (who could not be blamed for this colour change) reckoned she could 'save' them by boiling them in various solutions to remove the aberrant turquoise. She set about the task with gusto.

After several sessions in the washing machine, the trousers were passable. Not beige any more, but certainly not turquoise either. They were a very pale cream, almost all trace of any colour having been chemically erased. I reckoned that after a few clinics'-worth of scrabbling around on the floor of my consulting room and half a dozen mornings standing behind cows, the trousers would return to something like their original light brown. The biggest problem was that their paleness was exaggerated by a gentle hint of blue, which gave them a whiter-than-white appearance. 'Only for a few days, Julian,' I thought. 'They'll soon be back to normal brown rather than electric white.' Not being too concerned with fashion, Sue's comment about my dazzling trousers quickly left my head as I pored over the book, looking for a nice outside job, where the offending trousers would be covered up under waterproof leggings anyway.

But the only message left for me to deal with said: *Please phone Mrs Dill re Bertie and Bingo.*

Mrs Dill was an elderly lady who had kept Jack Russell terriers all her life. Her current two dogs were called Bertie and Bingo. They were brothers, at least in so far as they both had the same mother. Not even Mrs Dill could be sure whether or not they shared the same father. In any case, they were definitely related and had the relationship that one would expect of two sparring brothers. Bertie was the elder but his seniority in years didn't confer the respect he felt he deserved and the two dogs often got into skirmishes. I suspected this would be the problem today.

Mrs Dill was immaculately presented at all times, sporting an elegant coiffure of white hair and bright red lipstick, and she was always very pleasant. I tapped her number into the phone.

'Good morning, Mrs Dill. It's Julian here, from the vets. I'm just returning your call about the dogs. Is everything okay?'

'Oh, thank you so much, Julian. How very good of you to take the time to call me back,' she effused with the heavy lisp that made her voice so unmistakable. 'It's Bertie and Bingo. They've been at it again, you see. I gave them breakfast and, well, you know, they had a bit of a disagreement and Bertie has a hole in his neck and it's bleeding. There is blood all over Bingo and everything looks a terrible mess.'

'Okay, don't worry. Can you bring them down, Mrs Dill? I can have a look at them and sort them out. Are you all right?'

I knew that she would have tried to intervene to separate the two scrapping dogs and I knew that the paper-thin skin of an elderly lady would always come off much worse than that of the tough terriers. My own grandmother used to wade in, in just the same way, to break up skirmishes between various of the terriers she had throughout my childhood, and I remember the nasty purple bruises and angry puncture wounds that would be the result.

'Oh, Julian, how kind of you to ask! It's just a scratch on my arm. I am bleeding, but I'll survive. When would you like me to come down?'

'Straight away, if you can, Mrs Dill.'

The sooner I could get the bleeding wounds of the dogs cleaned and, if necessary, stitched up, the better.

'Oh, how very good of you. I'll be on my way. I shall just finish off my coffee. I'll be with you in about a quarter of an hour. I do hope that's all right.'

Mrs Dill was an amazing lady. In previous years she had spent each summer organizing and hosting the famous 'Jack Russell Tea Party'. This annual event, held in June, on the tiny cricket pitch in the grounds of Upsall Castle, just outside Thirsk, attracted national attention. It was, as the name suggested, a summer garden party where the only entry requirement was to bring a Jack Russell terrier. I had been to many similar garden parties whilst at university, where the invitation requested that guests bring not a Jack Russell, but a bottle of sparkling white wine or half a bottle of vodka. It was hard to say which summer garden party accoutrement would lead to a more lively afternoon — anyone who has known a Jack Russell would anticipate a riot when the dogs have the chance to mingle on the same cricket field on a warm summer day. Admittedly, there were often a few skirmishes, but the short-legged and wilful dogs usually got on together remarkably well and veterinary intervention was seldom necessary.

The dog owners would all bring picnics and there would be a dog show of sorts, with prizes for the most imaginative fancy dress, the best family of dogs, the prettiest bitch, the most handsome geriatric and so on. The dogs would love it, all standing especially proud as if realizing that they were on display.

Some years after she had retired from organizing the Jack Russell tea parties, Anne was chatting to Mrs Dill at a party (a normal one, without dogs).

'It's most irksome,' explained Mrs Dill. 'I have done an awful lot of good work in my time, raising money for charity and so on, but all I seem to be remembered for is organizing the Jack Russell Tea Party!'

She paused. 'But', she added, 'Jack Russells are simply the most wonderful of dogs.'

I checked through the notes of both Bertie and Bingo as I waited for Mrs Dill to arrive. The notes told the story of a pair of accident-prone dogs.

Bingo's notes read: *'Bingo has had a foul-smelling accident in the bathroom. Also deaf. Rubbing his head along the ground.'*

It was not clear whether the foul-smelling

accident and the deafness were thought to be connected.

Next: '*Bingo has taken to eating items of clothing, socks etc. Guts very active. Mrs D took decaying rabbit's ears off him this morning.*'

These kind of clinical notes were fairly typical for a wilful and confident but unthinking Jack Russell. They continued:

'*Bingo vomited five times this morning. Eaten some nylon stockings.*'

'*Bingo apparently has also eaten a Nurofen tablet this morning.*'

Bertie was less reckless with his dietary habits, but we saw him more regularly. His notes were more copious because he had a heart murmur and therefore needed regular checks. His weak heart was a relative term, as a Jack Russell with a bad heart is still a formidable force. It didn't stop him from fighting with his brother.

By the time I had finished perusing the notes of both dogs, Mrs Dill had arrived in the car park. From the window of my consulting room I watched her clambering out of the car clutching one of her dogs, who was covered in blood.

There was some remonstrating in the car park — the dog clearly did not want to attend the surgery that morning while there was unfinished business back in Upsall. Mrs Dill appeared only to have brought one of the dogs and he eventually trotted along beside the old lady, shaking his head as he walked. Even from a distance I could tell that it was Bertie, as his brown bits were paler than Bingo's, but on this occasion, most of his hair was pink and red after the fracas.

Nowadays, more of our time on the farm is spent looking after animals such as goats or alpacas. This Angora goat, kept for its fleece, is suffering from a badly broken leg. The fracture healed very well after the application of a fibreglass cast.

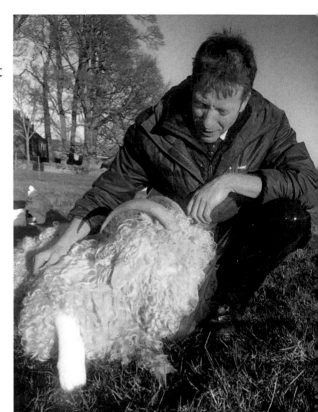

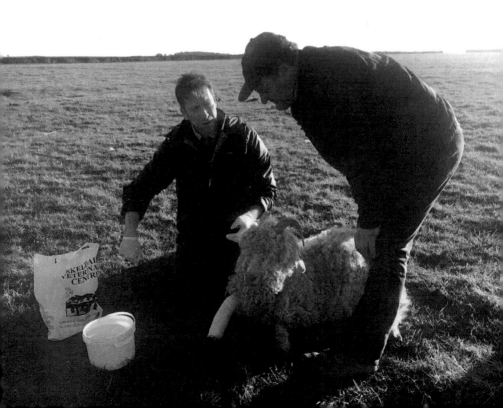

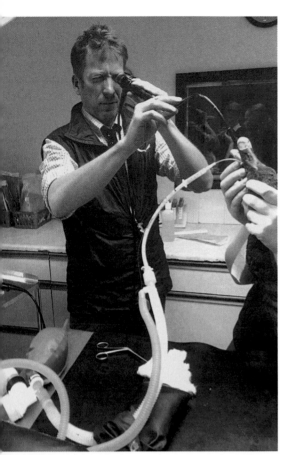

Left: This swan had been struggling to eat. Endoscopy allows us to look for things stuck down the throat. In this case I'm checking for fishing line.

Below: 'Hal', the Mangalitza boar, had just arrived from Holland. New breeding stock of this rare breed is hard to find. His arrival brought much-needed new genetics to the herd.

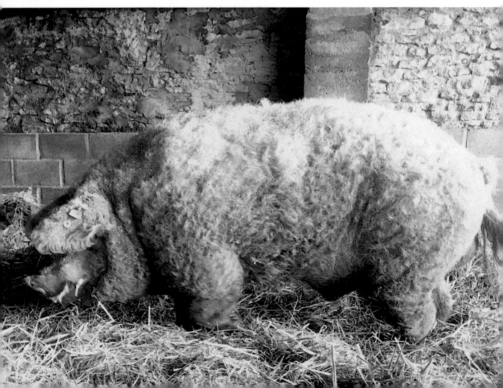

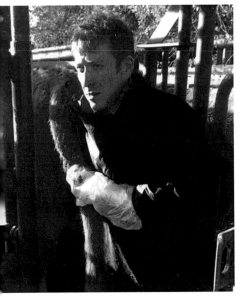

Left: Much of a large animal vet's time is spent behind the back end of a cow. In this case I am palpating inside the rectum to feel if the cow is pregnant. It's a standard job at the end of autumn.

Right and below: An early morning call, in the depths of winter, to help my young colleague Katy with a tough calving. The calf was a breech and it needed to be manipulated so it could be calved. It was an easy one for me, because all that was needed was some gentle reassurance and a bit of guidance. Katy is a very capable vet!

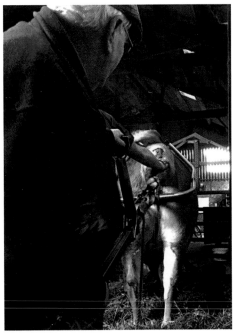

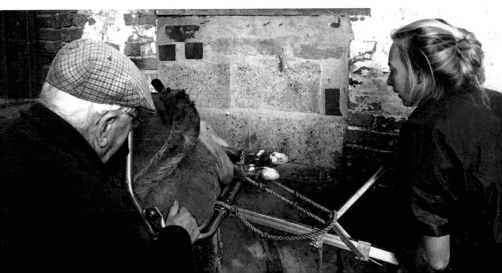

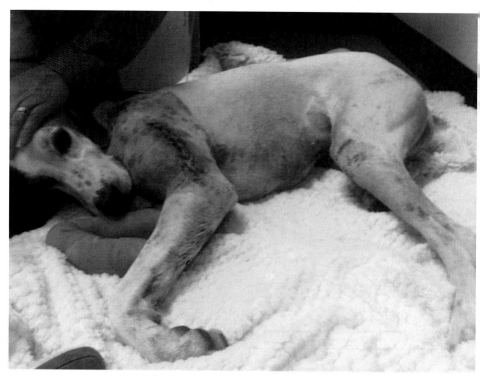

Penny was an amazing dog and extremely lucky. She looks very sorry for herself after the operation that took me into the small hours of the morning, but what a difference by the end of the summer!

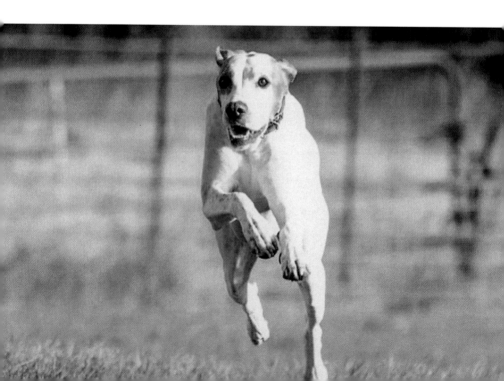

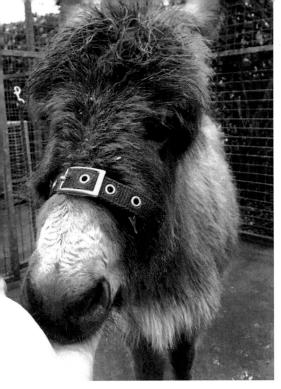

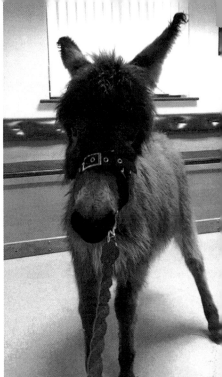

Archie, the miniature Mediterranean donkey, was a character. He had a retained testicle, which needed to be removed. About the same size as a Labrador, he made heads turn in the waiting room of my practice. The anaesthetic and surgery was performed on the floor. Sarah, my colleague who is very good with equine work, performed the operation.

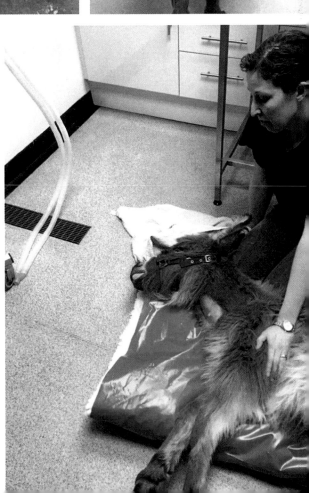

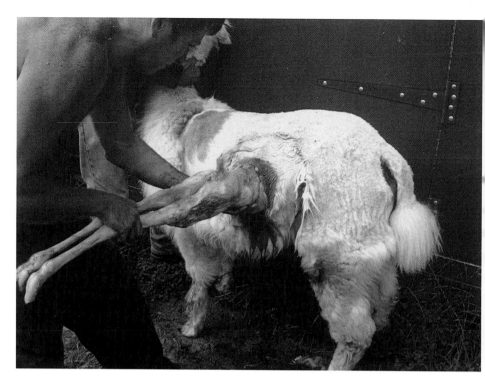

My very first alpaca caesarean was photographed by farmer Linda McDonald, a keen photographer and a good friend. Hers was the first farm in the area to get alpacas so it was a steep learning curve for everyone. The mother and baby cria did very well and I followed the progress of them both for many years.

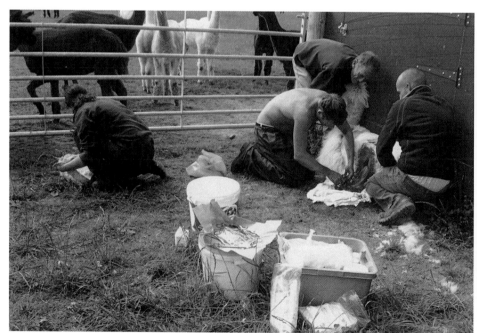

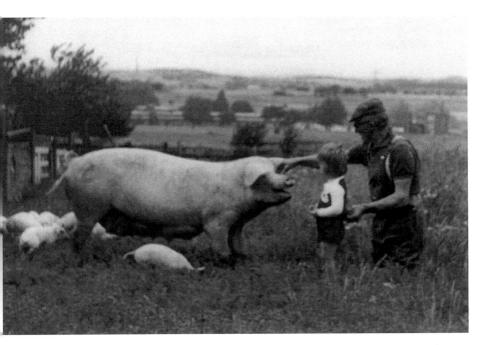

Above: This is one of the first pictures of me with the animals that would become such a big part of my life. My Grandfather, Jack Taylor, shows me his best sow. It's hard to tell what I think of it, but I do have many memories of my first experiences with animals.

Below: Posing with a cute lamb for a photo shoot. Who would have thought I would ever be doing this?

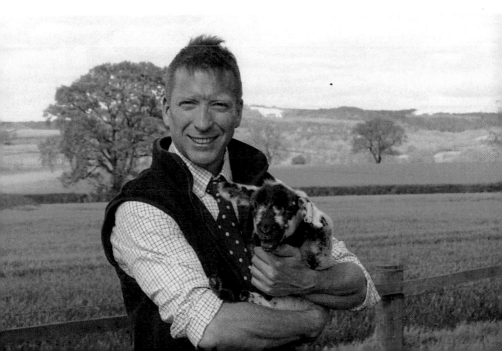

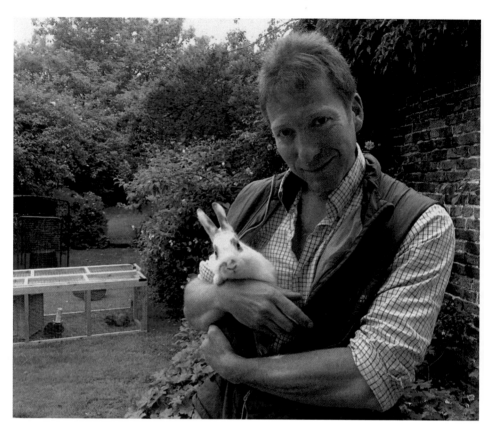

Luna (above), and Sparkle and Shine (below): My family's collection of small and furry pets. They are wonderful little creatures and all get along brilliantly.

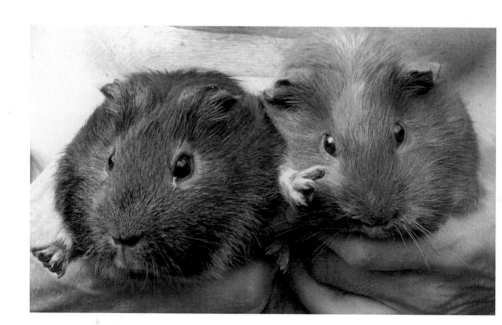

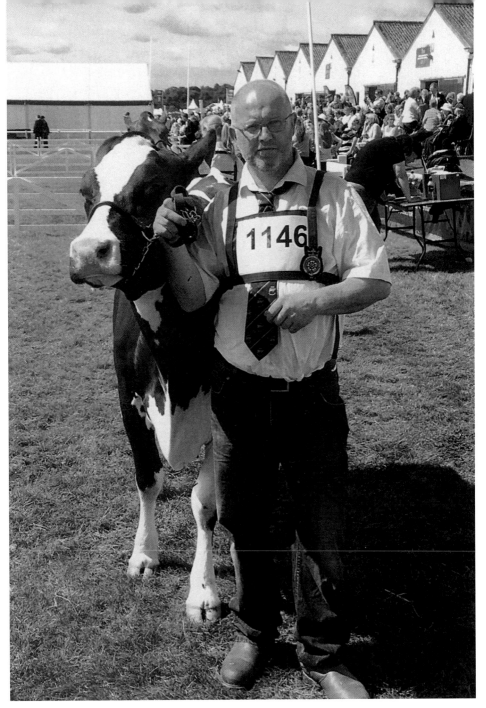

Martin Jackson has become a great friend over the last few years and he has a small herd of dairy shorthorn cattle. His aim is to follow in his uncle's footsteps and win the top prize at the Great Yorkshire Show. It wasn't to be this particular year, but he is, quite rightly, very proud of his lovely cow.

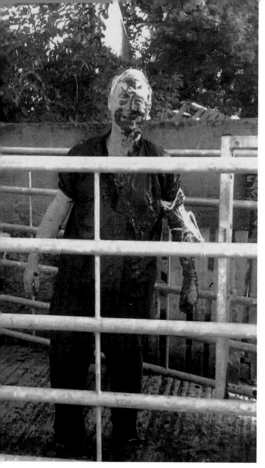

Left: My colleague Peter, with whom I have had some great experiences, is in the wrong place at the wrong time. A coughing cow with loose faeces is a dangerous combination. Peter must have either been out of practice, or too slow to get out of the way!

Below: One of my all time favourite places, Gormire, with Whitestonecliffe behind. It is just as beautiful in midwinter as at any other time of the year and it is always so peaceful and tranquil.

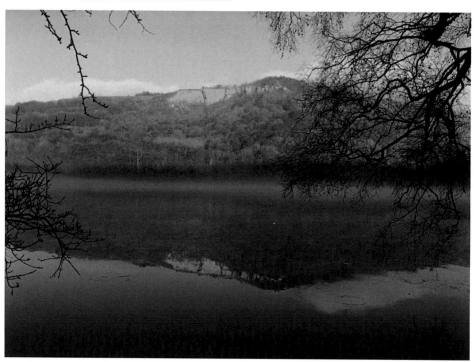

Right: Kneepads the goat was always in trouble. You can just tell it from his mischievous expression!

Below: A perfect way to start a Sunday on call! The calf was way too big for this heifer and she needed a caesarean. Perfect facilities made this a straightforward procedure. The calf was on its feet before I left and I was home in time for breakfast.

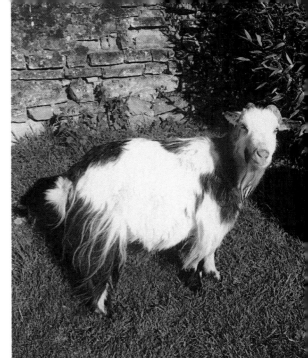

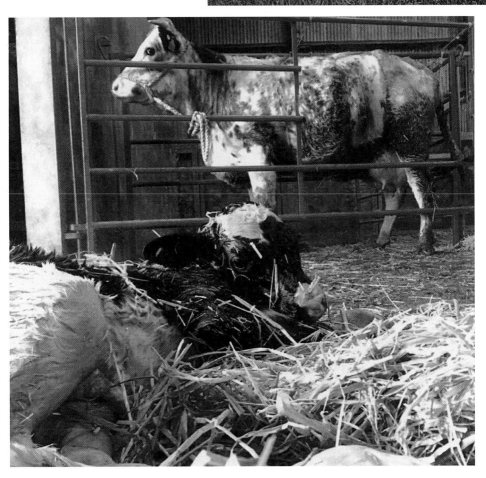

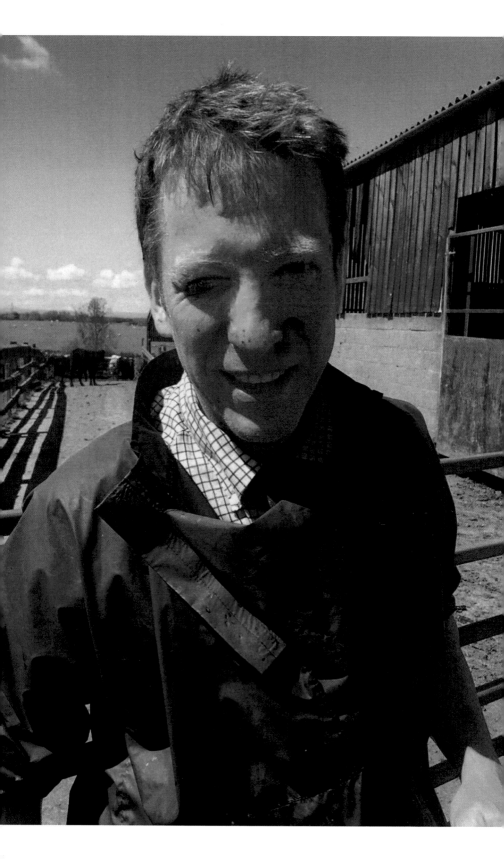

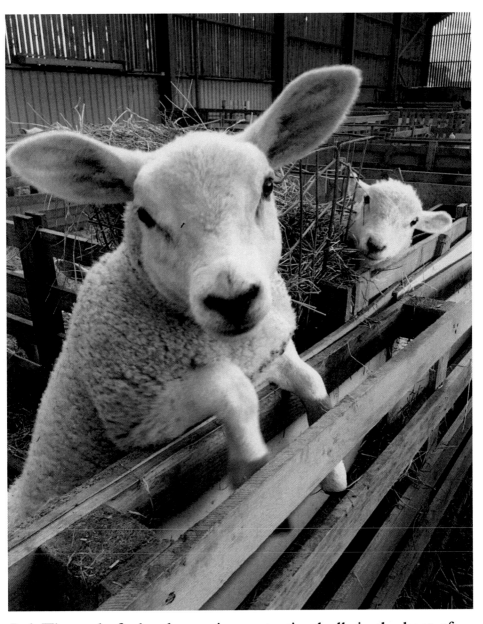

Left: The end of a hard morning castrating bulls in the heat of midsummer. Being wrapped up in plastic is not great when it is very hot. My shirt was sopping wet with sweat and the blood and antibiotic spray has left plenty of marks – at least I escaped without any injuries!

Above: 'Lamby' was one of my most challenging cases, suffering from a terrible ruptured rectal prolapse. I was sure she wouldn't survive the emergency surgery, but sure enough, this is her three months later at her farm in Dewsbury.

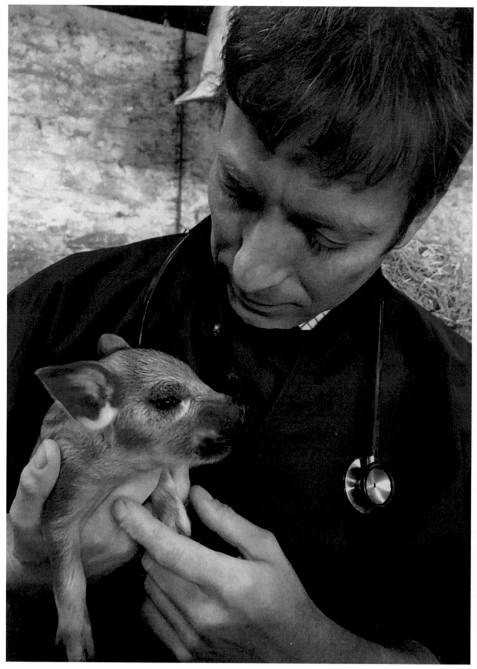
A baby piglet called Tiny Tim receiving a health check. This one is a rare swallowbelly Mangalitza piglet and proves to be very healthy.

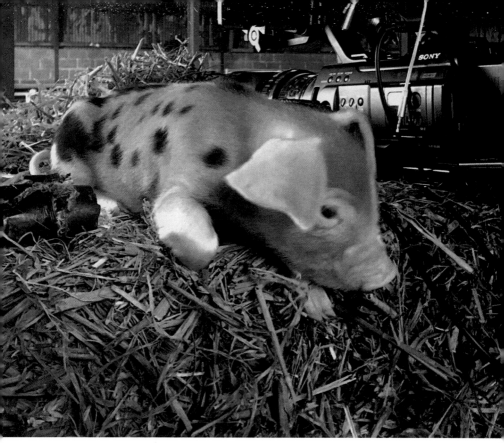

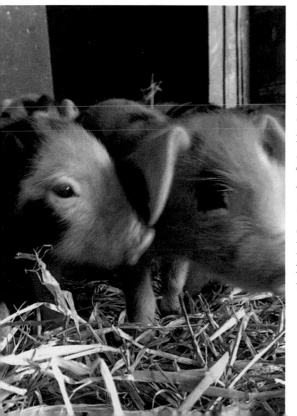

On a return visit to a smallholding to check up on a case, the camera crew is never far away. The camera is quickly put down to make space for cuddling baby piglets. These are Elsie's babies: the result of Chris and my exploits earlier that summer. I felt like a proud father when I came to visit.

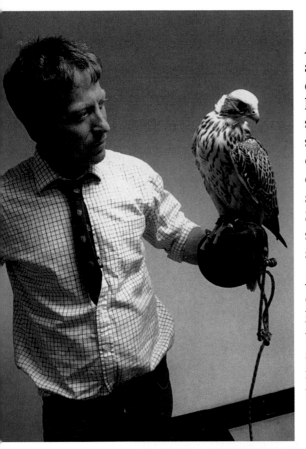

Left: This gyrfalcon was an unusual visitor to my evening clinic. It is the largest of the falcon species and beautiful to see at close quarters. This one needs nothing more complicated than to have a microchip implanted. Some days we do literally see All Creatures Great and Small.

Below: It's hard to beat checking over young kittens. Even though these two inquisitive creatures are from the same litter, it is amazing how different they both look.

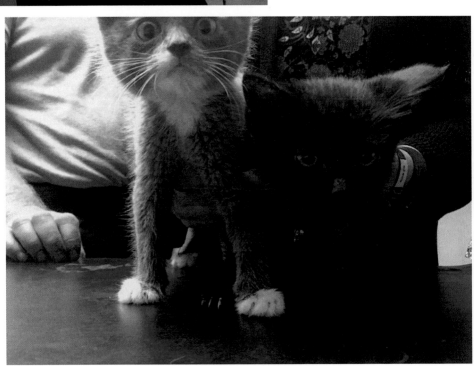

I met Mrs Dill and Bertie in the waiting room. Before I could say hello and usher the pair into the consulting room, Mrs Dill, with her customary enthusiasm, stopped in her tracks, stared at me and gushed, 'Oh, how simply splendid, Julian! I do like to see a man dressed in smart white trousers!'

She was obviously even more impressed by my attire than Sue had been earlier, but her lisp made her proclamation seem even more ridiculous. She could hardly have constructed a sentence with more 'S's in it!

Once they were in my room, I lifted Bertie onto the table, without any objection from him at all, and started my examination. There was, as Mrs Dill had correctly identified, a puncture wound in Bertie's neck and blood all over him. The laceration was quite deep — as deep as a terrier's canine tooth is long — and about an inch long, gaping open like the mouth of a fish. There was also a small tear in Bertie's left ear. I explained that I would need to sedate Bertie to clean up his injuries and put a couple of sutures in the gaping wound. Often bite wounds are left open so infection doesn't get trapped under the skin, but if the wound is large and gaping and if we can do the surgery promptly before infection takes hold, the healing process is speeded up.

The small cut to Bertie's ear also needed attention. It was very small but these little nicks can produce copious amounts of blood. A bit of blood goes a long way on a white dog, but a lot of blood goes much further, and this was the reason why Bertie was a shade of strawberry

151

pink. I explained my plan to Mrs Dill, who was delighted that I could repair the wounds so promptly. I took Bertie into the prep room to give him a sedative, which would take a few minutes to work, and then returned to my consulting room where Mrs Dill was waiting.

'Shall I have a look at your arm?' I offered.

'Oh, how kind. It's just a small scratch, but there is plenty of blood!' she commented. 'I did try to stop the boys from fighting, but they were just so determined. I couldn't really help.'

The wound was not deep, but there was some bruising developing, extending in both directions along her forearm. I wiped the dried blood off with some antiseptic and then applied a light dressing. Mrs Dill seemed very appreciative and continued her profuse thanks.

Bertie was swiftly sorted out in theatre and was happy to see his owner as I brought him back to the waiting room. He was stitched up, his bloody war wounds were cleaned and he looked not much the worse for his morning's exploits. The same could not be said for my poor trousers, which were now bluish cream with large red smears of blood from both patient and owner. They were destined for another appointment with the washing machine, very shortly.

Later that day, after evening surgery had finished, I was relating the story of the dogs and Mrs Dill's admiration of my trousers to Tim, one of my senior colleagues. It seemed her liking for a man in white was long-standing. Tim recalled having a similar conversation with Mrs Dill many years earlier. It was in the corridor of the old surgery at 23, Kirkgate — the original practice from which Alf Wight, better known as James Herriot, worked. In those days, veterinary surgeons wore white coats, just like doctors, pharmacists and pretty much all other healthcare professionals. Tim was wearing his white coat over a pale checked shirt and even paler, faded-once-beige trousers. As he rounded the corner from his consulting room and headed to the waiting room to call his next patient, Tim was greeted with the same compliment from Mrs Dill: 'Oh, how smart! All in white!'

On that particular day, Mrs Dill had brought her dog, not a Jack Russell this time, but a little Pekinese, to see Mr Sinclair. Donald Sinclair was the larger-than-life senior partner of the practice, upon whom the character of Siegfried Farnon was based in the Herriot books. Like many old veterinary senior partners, his retirement was long overdue and his eyesight wasn't as good as it had been. After an examination and the appropriate injection of penicillin, Mrs Dill went back to reception and joined the queue to pay. When she got to the desk and opened her handbag to get out her purse, she was surprised to find the handbag full of oily white antibiotic solution. The Pekinese had not received a drop of the medicine!

'Oh my goodness! I have penicillin in my bag!' she said with surprise but, unswervingly dignified and polite, she paid her bill, arranged her next appointment and left the practice, unperturbed by the blatant mistake. Apparently, the dog made a full recovery.

The Mystery of the Floppy Heifers

'Can you come and have a look, Julian? I had one of your young vets out on Sunday, but this heifer's still not right, and there's another one out in the field that looks like it's heading the same way.'

I could tell from the tone of Robert's voice that he was worried about his heifer. He was a very experienced farmer and had seen most of the diseases and problems that faced both dairy cows and their calves. He would usually give me a diagnosis before I arrived on Mowbray Farm, but today was different.

I confirmed that I would be with him as soon as I had finished afternoon surgery, but first I needed to speak with Laura, my colleague who had treated the heifer the previous Sunday. The animal had been in one of the sheds. Robert had brought her inside on the Saturday because she looked poorly — lying down when all the other animals were standing up — but, Laura explained, there was not much to go on.

'To be honest,' she said with a frown, 'I couldn't find a lot wrong with her, other than that she was lying down and wouldn't stand up. I gave her some calcium, some anti-inflammatories and multivitamins and said to call back with a progress report. I was hoping you'd be able to have a look at her, actually, because I don't really know what to do next.'

It was a frank and honest assessment that left me without many clues. Being a veterinary surgeon is like being a detective. As well as carrying out our clinical examination, we have to quiz the owner in detail to gain as much information as possible about the behaviour of the animal, its environment, its diet and its demeanour. Hopefully, from all this, and with the help of laboratory tests and imaging, we can then make a tentative diagnosis. In farm animals, diagnosis can be even more difficult. Clinical examination may yield less information because of the large size of the animal and, sadly, financial constraints often limit how many laboratory tests can be undertaken. For farmers trying to scrape a living from their stock, a test that costs more than the value of the animal is often not a feasible proposition (unless, of course, there are implications for the whole herd). This afternoon, I had the feeling that I was going to have to draw on my years of experience as much as anything else.

When I arrived, I found the heifer lying down, with her head lolling to one side. Her mentation didn't seem quite as sharp as it should have been and she moved her head slowly, as if she had a headache. The first thing to do was to perform a thorough clinical examination. This was certainly going to be a diagnostic challenge.

Her temperature was slightly elevated at 102.8°F. This was a starting point, but not a tremendously helpful one. A sky-high temperature always means infection in a cow, and if we find this at the beginning of our examination, everything else is straightforward. A slightly increased temperature *might* indicate an infection, but not necessarily — so no certainty so far. When I listened to her rumen with my stethoscope, the contractions sounded weak. Her lungs were clear, rectal examination was normal, her reflexes were normal and her legs seemed to work okay. I felt sure she *could* stand if she had the urge or the impetus.

I questioned Robert, trying to identify what might have triggered the problem. She was one of a batch of about thirty yearling heifers out at grass in an established pasture, not heavily fertilized. They had been there for about four weeks, hadn't been moved recently and were just eating the grass without any supplementary feed. They had been wormed and vaccinated with the usual things. There was one other heifer with drooping ears, who didn't look quite right. She was still in the field, which was about two miles away, with the rest of the group. There were absolutely no clues and no predisposing factors.

The only thing I could come up with that vaguely fitted with the signs was a condition called thromboembolic meningoencephalitis. This is a disease caused by a bacterium called Haemophilus somnus that usually causes pneumonia (the name has now been changed to Histophilus somnus, but it's hard to get the name you originally learnt at university out of your head). On occasions it can lodge in the brain of a young bovine and cause a condition that is also known as 'sleeper sickness' because it makes affected cattle look as if they are asleep. The disease usually affects housed cattle rather than those out in an airy, grass field but otherwise the signs fitted.

I administered an intravenous antibiotic of a type that would cross the blood-brain barrier and therefore reach any bacteria in the heifer's brain. I also gave her a strong painkiller to fix the presumed headache, then explained to Robert that I would need to come and repeat the process the next day. After this, Robert climbed into his tractor and I followed him in my Mitsubishi, to the field where the rest of the group were grazing. I wanted to see the other animals, particularly the one with the drooping ears that was causing Robert concern, in the hope that this would provide me with more of an idea about what might be going on.

The route to the field wound between two hedgerows that were bursting with colour from the wild geraniums and cow parsley that spilt over onto the track. It wasn't muddy, but the deep ruts were baked dry, making it much more suited to a tractor than my four-by-four. I bounced along the track, blissfully unaware that it was a journey with which I would become very familiar over the next few weeks.

The bunch of heifers looked pretty normal, standing in the field, grazing. We leant on the gate and studied the animals but neither of us could see one with drooping ears and, after a quarter of an hour of scrutiny, I felt happy that there were none showing any similar signs.

Robert said he would stay for a while, but after arranging a time to re-examine the affected heifer the following day, I waved goodbye.

Twenty-four hours later I was back, repeating my perfunctory tests on the heifer, who looked a bit better. She was standing up and had drunk some water, but her head was still well and truly pointing into the corner of her pen, and she was still showing no interest in her surroundings. Her temperature was now back to normal, so I repeated the same treatment with cautious optimism. Haemophilus somnus cases usually take several doses of antibiotics before they show any sign of recovery, and some don't respond at all, so it was still early days for this treatment.

Robert told me that he had spent half an hour watching the cattle in the field after I had left and he had been back there again this morning, but had seen nothing suspicious. I knew he would have been watching them like a hawk. Again, I made arrangements to return the following day to give another intravenous dose to the poorly heifer, then headed back to do battle with a clinic full of dogs and cats.

The next day, Robert phoned the surgery just as I was getting ready to set off to his farm. He was very worried.

'Julian, there are another three heifers that do not look right. I think they've got the same thing. One is quite bad-like and the other two not as bad, but there's sommat up with them. I thought I should let you know 'cos you might need to bring more bottles of stuff to inject them wi'.'

When I arrived, the sight in the pen was a sorry one. Four yearling heifers were in the large pen, out of place because on a hot, dry summer day like today these animals should have been grazing in a grassy paddock. One, my first case, was standing, staring into the same corner as she had been the previous day. She looked pretty much the same. The optimist in me said that she looked a little brighter, but the realist was telling me that she was not progressing as well as I would have hoped. The other three animals were all lying down and one — the worst — had its head curled around as if it was looking at its flank, trying to go to sleep.

I examined them all. Two of the new cases were not too bad and leapt to their feet when I went up to them. They were soon trying to escape, so we ushered them, one at a time, into the cattle crush so I could check them over. The worst one, though, made no attempt to stand up. Again, no specific signs were evident when I examined the animals, and the clinical picture still looked more like Haemophilus somnus than anything else, but I still had a nagging feeling we might be missing something. It was time to take some blood samples to try to reach a definitive diagnosis.

Robert was happy with this and, even though it would add an extra hundred pounds or so to the bill, we both knew it was the best thing to do. I returned from my car with a handful of vacutainer tubes and took a blood sample from the tail vein of each of the heifers. I treated all the animals with antibiotics again, and headed straight to the veterinary laboratory in Thirsk, where I could hand in the samples. It was always useful to grab a quick chat with one of the pathologists when we called in at the lab on our way back to the practice. On this day, though, no one was available, which was a shame because I could have really done with their thoughts. I would have to save the conversation for when the blood results were back, in a two or three days' time.

It was an anxious wait. I made a couple more visits to see Robert and to check the rest of the heifers in the pen. I also went back to the field, on my own, each lunchtime to look out for other early cases and to scour the hedgerows for anything that might be causing the problem. Any clues that I could find must surely be helpful. I searched for poisonous plants, as there are a few that can cause peculiar illnesses in cattle. I also poked about in the hedge bottoms for old batteries (used to power electric fences) or rusting old metal, which could have been covered with poisonous lead paint. Lead poisoning can cause neurological disease in cattle, although it is usually manifested by blindness and the heifers' signs didn't really fit.

When the results finally came chugging out of the fax machine, I was crestfallen. All four samples were negative for Haemophilus. I called the lab.

Gary, the duty vet, explained that this negative result would tend to rule out the disease, although a definitive diagnosis could only be made (as all good pathologists always tell us) by a post mortem examination of an affected brain. Gary assured me that this would give the certain answer. The only problem was, none of the animals were dead.

I immediately called Robert to tell him the results of the blood tests and to discuss Gary's suggestion. It was obvious what must happen next and Robert agreed that we should euthanase the worst-affected animal. The next morning, though, standing in the pen in which I had spent more time recently than anywhere else, the decision did not feel so easy to make. It felt as if we were giving up on whichever poor animal we chose, and it was even more frustrating because we had put so much time, care and emotional energy into trying to save the heifers, not to mention all the drugs I had given them.

I phoned Gary, to tell him that a carcass would be with him within an hour. The worst part was choosing which animal to sacrifice. We both felt like judge and jury as we perused the pen of sick heifers, deciding which was the one least likely to survive. At this time, the first heifer was stoically surviving, although she still spent much of her time staring at the wall, occasionally putting her head in the bucket of water that Robert would offer her, or nibbling on the pile of silage nearby. One of the new cases — the heifer with her head lolling against her side — was certainly the most serious and this was the one that we picked. I drew up a big syringe of the drug used for euthanasia, knowing that it was unlikely that I would actually need the full fifty millilitres that I had loaded, as she was so weak. Whilst it felt wrong to pick any one of the patients, it was in fact, probably the kindest thing to do — she was very poorly and clearly suffering.

As I predicted, she didn't need the full syringe. Within five minutes the back door of the trailer was closed and Robert was taking the animal to the lab for an appointment with Gary.

Gary must have worked through his lunch break, because I got a call midway through afternoon surgery with the results of the first part of the post mortem examination.

'Hello, Julian!'

Gary's tone sounded optimistic, but as it turned out, it was only the excited voice of a pathologist in action.

'There's absolutely nothing to see in this heifer. No lesions at all, I'm afraid. Nothing to go on. Of course, we will be doing histology on the brain, CSF cytology and immuno-histopathology on the brain and meninges, just to be sure. Then there is toxicology on the liver, kidneys and what-not. That'll take a week or so, I'm afraid. Some of it needs to go to Weybridge, you see. So far, not a sausage.'

The phrases 'and whatnot' and 'not a sausage' seemed utterly incongruous amongst all the other technical terminology, but I knew what Gary meant. I also knew what this meant for my chances of a speedy diagnosis and my chances of stopping the progression of the herd's illness. I was no further forward.

Gary continued, 'Is there any chance that it could be lead poisoning?'

'I've been all around the field and can't find anything at all, Gary,' I replied, miserably. 'It's a pretty bare pasture and nothing toxic. Certainly nothing that I could see, anyway.'

'Let me think about it, Julian. I'll get back to you after I've had more time to think. Meantime, we'll wait for the next results.'

And with that, Gary went off the phone and back to his post mortem samples.

Gloomily, I put down the receiver, only to pick it up again to relay the unhelpful news to Robert.

He was even gloomier than I was, as I spoke to him on his mobile. He was standing in the field of heifers, where yet more were sick, ears and head drooping downwards. Worse still, two of the initial batch had died despite the injections that we had been giving. Put off by the negative results that I had just passed on, Robert was not keen on sending these two carcasses to be tested. At this point sending samples to the lab seemed to be a fruitless and expensive pastime.

After a day or so of waiting for Gary and his histology results, the situation at Mowbray Farm had not improved. A handful of new cases had appeared. A couple of the early cases seemed to be rallying slowly, but nothing dramatic. The next phone call from the lab delivered more negative results. The histology of the brain had ruled out my presumed diagnosis of Haemophilus.

'I'll come and have a look at the farm, if you'd like, Julian,' offered Gary. 'Two heads are better than one.'

We arranged to meet the next day. It is the sign of a serious situation when a ministry vet leaves his office and reaches for his immaculate Wellington boots, and I was glad of any extra input that he could offer.

Gary followed me to the farm and donned his spotless wellies and virginal, white waterproof overall. I showed him the sad collection of dopey heifers in the shed. He asked all the same questions that I had asked to Robert, who must have been sick of repeating the same answers over and over again. Then he reached for his stethoscope and pulled out his thermometer. Now, I know a bit about stethoscopes. I use one many times a day. There are two types. The good ones have ends made of brushed aluminium, with thick, flexible, rubber pipes and snug earpieces that make it easy to listen to the subtle sounds that signify life and health in our patients. The other type is often handed out free with a drug order or a consignment of dog food, and is more suitable for a child's play set than as an aid to diagnosis. It was the latter that Gary used to examine some of the heifers. I could tell that his examination was not particularly detailed, but this did not matter because, as he pulled his plastic stethoscope from his ears, he declared his diagnosis with aplomb.

'I think this is a case of botulinum poisoning,' he announced.

I was surprised by the assurance with which he had reached this conclusion. I had always associated botulism with cattle eating dirty or contaminated silage, or animals drinking from a muddy, duck-infested pond. The field was bone dry and the water came from a water trough. I'd checked this — it was clean and the water was fresh, coming as it did from a nearby spring. The

164

cattle had not eaten any silage for about two months. I could not imagine how on earth the herd could have been exposed to botulism. I also remembered from my university days that achieving a proper diagnosis was very difficult. To test for the disease we would need to take a sample from one of the dead heifers and inject it into mice, to see if they died of botulism. This was not a palatable idea and was certainly not going to happen if I had anything to do with it. It was true, though, that botulism caused neuro-muscular paralysis and would result in weak cattle, reluctant or unable to stand. It could look like this outbreak. As I understood it, the mortality level would be very high and affected cattle would succumb very quickly. Anyone familiar with 'botox' injections into a wrinkled face is aware of the muscular paralysis that occurs. Gary was suggesting that this effect was occurring on a grand scale.

'Let's go and have a look at the paddock,' Gary suggested.

'Do you use poultry manure as fertilizer?' he asked Robert as we clambered into our respective vehicles to embark on the bumpy ride down the flower-lined track to the field.

'We have used it in the past on the arable land, but not on this field,' confirmed Robert.

'Do you know if there is any of it piled up, nearby? Maybe that other farmers are using?'

'Not that I know of.' Robert looked as perplexed as I was by this new line of questioning.

Once we got to the field, surrounded by its

sparce hedge of hawthorn and oak trees, Gary was like a terrier, rummaging into rabbit holes and peering into the water troughs, looking for clues.

I scuttled along behind him, not really sure what he was looking for. His fervour reminded me of the French police inspector in one of my kids' favourite films, *Madagascar 3: Europe's Most Wanted*, as she searched for the missing zoo animals. He wasn't exactly sniffing on all fours, but very nearly, such was his enthusiasm for the task in hand.

His trail led us to the edge of the field and over a ditch, thick with brambles and wild roses, but the spikes did not impede the ministry vet. He caught sight of something in the distance, at the edge of a field about a quarter of a mile away, and nearly broke into a run.

'Look, Julian! It's a mound of poultry manure! Follow me!' he exclaimed.

As we rustled along, me in my waterproof trousers and Gary in his white ministry-issue protective suit, he explained his theory.

'You see, this is what happens — that pile of poultry manure is from the bottom of a broiler shed, where chickens are reared for Sunday roasts. The manure is a brilliant fertilizer and farmers get it to dress their land. The problem is, if any chickens die, they get trampled into the manure and their dead bodies partially decompose.'

His manner was so matter-of-fact.

'Since these birds hardly ever receive antibiotics in their food, the dead chickens decompose quickly and botulinum bacteria grow within them. The toxin builds up to quite high levels,' he explained.

This still didn't explain why the field of heifers, about a quarter of a mile away and separated by a hedge, might have been contaminated by the toxin. I was sure none of the heifers would have escaped the field to have a quick chicken snack.

'Then it's the foxes, you see,' Gary continued. 'They come along and dig in the manure, looking for bits of chicken.'

I still could not understand how this affected my heifers, but he went on: 'They grab the chicken bits and pull them back to their den to feed their young. Foxes being foxes, they usually take more than they can carry, so they will drop bits of chicken carcass en route. Cattle do not usually eat this sort of thing but — and this is the key — if the grass is very short *like it is now* they might be tempted to sniff or nibble on a bit of dead chicken. They are so sensitive to botulinum toxin, even a tiny bit can cause illness.'

It sounded like the way a disease would be spread in the drought-affected savannahs of Africa, but now, it seemed, it was happening in North Yorkshire!

By this time, we had arrived at the brown mound of smelly, flaky poultry poo and Gary was already standing on top. Within just a few moments he had discovered several little holes where something — we presumed a fox — had been scrabbling, digging for food. With imagination it was even possible to see tiny fox footprints extending from the hole that had been dug.

Gary didn't shout out the words 'ta dah!' as he stood at the top of his mound, where he was doing a great impression of being the king of the castle, but he might as well have done. We could not prove his theory, but it sounded plausible and he seemed certain he was correct.

As he leapt from foot to foot in his enthusiasm, Gary went on to explain: 'We see this all the time now. It's ever since poultry farmers stopped using antibiotics to promote the growth of their chickens. It's good for chickens and people but bad for cattle if they accidentally eat the bones. The dead chickens are just full of botulism, you see. We've seen half a dozen cases this year, over the whole of the north of England.'

The mystery appeared to have been solved. We explained it to an astonished Robert, and suggested moving the cattle to another field, well away from the offending pile of poultry muck. There was no effective treatment for the animals which were suffering — all my visits and injections were for nothing — but at least we had a diagnosis, could remove the cause and prevent sorry episodes like this happening again.

Once the move had taken place, no more cases developed. The statistics for the outbreak were bad, though — eight out of forty-one animals died, eight affected animals recovered, twenty-five were, thankfully, unaffected. The muck was spread and Robert and I, despite having many more wrinkles than we did before the episode, swore that neither of us would ever visit a beauty salon for a botox injection as long as we lived!

Lady Anne and the Colt with Colic

The small village of Sutton-under-Whitestone-cliffe takes its name from the imposing limestone escarpment that dominates the skyline to the east of Thirsk. The cliff marks the beginning of the North York Moors National Park and it always gives me a thrill when I have the chance to negotiate the steep hairpin bend near its summit. On the edge of this village was where Lady Anne kept her young stallions.

Lady Anne was a frail, elderly lady who lived alone in a small, messy, 1970s bungalow that looked very out of place in the picturesque village. A visit to her stables always sounded like an idyllic way to spend a sunny morning. Nothing was further from the truth though, because Lady Anne owned a couple of brood mares and a collection of very unruly yearlings, all bred out of these ageing mares. Whilst Lady Anne had obviously been a force to be reckoned with in her youth — the photographs around her living room were testament to her formidable equine background — she was, when I knew her during my first few years at Skeldale, finding it a challenge to manage her animals.

So, the call to see a yearling with colic at Sutton Stables on this misty summer morning was always going to be one for the junior vet. As

I packed up all the extra bits of equipment that I might need — a bottle of liquid paraffin, a selection of sedatives and painkillers and a stomach tube — some additional instructions from the senior partner issued forth from the vets' office: 'Make sure you get a cheque from her. She owes us a fortune! It's like pulling teeth trying to get money from her! She's not paid anything off her account for over six months.'

'Great!' I thought. As if the clinical part of this morning's job wasn't going to be hard enough, I had the job of debt collecting, too. That was not something for which vet school had prepared me!

I had one final check of my car boot, just to make sure everything was there, and took a deep breath before embarking on the ten-minute journey towards Sutton Bank. Mist was clinging stubbornly to the fields despite the increasing intensity of the midsummer sun. It would soon evaporate and the haze would give way to the strong June heat. Whilst it was a glorious day, I was not looking forward to the job ahead of me.

Lady Anne usually packaged her mares off to stud in the spring then, once they were pregnant, she would have them back for the summer to graze, quietly gestating their foals. Just before the foals were due to be born, the mares would return to the stud, where they would get expert and constant supervision by specialized staff and veterinary surgeons, who dealt with nothing else. So specialist is the job of an equine stud vet, that once the UK stud season is over, they often travel to New Zealand, where the stud season is in the opposite half of the year, so that they are dealing with breeding animals all year round. Soon after Lady Anne's mares gave birth, they would be mated again and return to Sutton, pregnant once more with a foal at foot. It was Lady Anne's job to nurture and rear these foals and supervise their progression into sensible, well-handled and well-mannered youngsters before they were sent to a racehorse trainer, to be honed for glorious success at Cheltenham or Aintree.

The system worked well, except for the fact that Lady Anne was now in her eighties. Judging by the slowness of her movement, her permanent reliance on a walking stick and her general frailty, she had enough of a challenge looking after herself, let alone half a dozen young horses.

I parked my car by the stables and, as I waited for her to arrive from her bungalow, I peered into each box, looking for my patient, but all were empty. It was several minutes before she tottered out of the side door, terribly stooped and very precarious on her legs.

'Oh, it's you, is it?' was the terse greeting from the old lady, when she finally made it to the stables. She did not look delighted to see me.

'Hello, Lady Anne. How are you?' I replied.

'Not very good. My knees are knackered and my back is bloody awful. And this yearling is bad, too. He's been like it since first thing this morning. I could see him from my bedroom window, you see?'

'How is he to handle, Lady Anne?' I asked, suspecting I already knew the answer.

'He's not really very good to handle at all,' she confirmed.

My heart began to sink.

'He's quite a strong yearling, you know. Well, he's actually a two-year-old, but I still think of him as a yearling. I haven't really had much chance to handle him — not as much as I would have liked. It's my knees, you see. He's out here, in the paddock next to the house, I'll show you.'

She pointed in the direction I needed to head, as if suggesting that I go first. She knew I could walk quicker than her. When I rounded the corner, my already sinking heart sank as far as it would go. The horse was rolling around in the middle of the paddock, obviously in a great deal of pain. It was clearly a very bad case of colic and was going to be every bit as difficult to manage as I had expected.

Colic is the term used to describe abdominal pain in any animal. Horses are particularly prone to colic, because they have such an enormously long intestine. A cow uses its rumen to digest the cellulose in grass and therefore bovine intestines are not as long. Horses, like rabbits, rely on their huge hindgut to do the same job as a cow's rumen. The great length that is required for this purpose means that the bowel can easily get twisted or pulled into the wrong place, a bit like an unravelled ball of string. This leads to stretching or distension, which is very painful and in some cases can be very serious. A horse with colic will kick at its belly and roll around on the floor, writhing in agony. Sometimes this rolling can make things much worse as the mass of guts can twist further.

The cause of the pain can be relatively simple. Spasmodic, colic, for example, where the intestines contract vigorously often for no obvious reason or cause, can be very painful but is easy to treat with the correct drugs. An impacted colic can be equally painful and is caused by a partial blockage of the large intestines, by hard faeces, soil, sand or matted-together grass. This usually occurs at a sharp bend in the colon called the pelvic flexure, and needs to be treated with large volumes of laxative, administered by nasogastric tube. It works well, but requires a rectal examination to make the diagnosis, followed by the successful passing of a stomach tube up the horse's nose, which then needs to be held in place for about ten minutes whilst a couple of litres of mineral oil are funnelled down. As we both peered at the writhing youngster in the middle of the paddock, I sincerely hoped this was not what we were dealing with today. I didn't relish the prospect of inserting my arm into one end of the horse or a pipe into the other.

The most serious type of colic occurs when part of the bowel twists and becomes entrapped. These cases are very dangerous for the horse and can only be treated by surgical correction by an equine surgeon. Add in conditions like grass sickness, which causes colic by virtue of the intestines becoming paralysed, and conditions that masquerade as colic, such as 'choke', and you can see that working out exactly what is happening inside the abdomen of an affected horse can be a diagnostic challenge. It is difficult enough in a calm, quiet patient, but in an unhandled colt, rolling around on the grass in the middle of a field, it was going to be ten times more challenging.

'At least he'll be easy to catch,' I thought.

Often horses turned out in summer fields are not keen on being caught, especially by a stranger smelling of surgical spirit and other animals. There was no way Lady Anne could do it, though, so between rolls, and whilst avoiding the flailing legs of the youngster, I managed to loop the lead rope round his neck and steady him down. Before long, with some gentle coercion, I had the front part of the head collar over his nose and then the strap behind his ears so I could buckle it up. It was clear, however, that I could not progress further without giving him a hefty dose of sedative and I kicked myself for not bringing it with me in my pocket. I would have to leave Lady Anne in charge while I went back to the car.

'I'll take him now,' said the old lady, without hesitation. She was very confident with horses and this colt obviously had a little more respect for his owner than I gave him credit for. They were used to each other's company, after all.

'That's a good boy, Trevor,' she reassured her horse. It seemed an incongruous name for such a handsome and headstrong beast. He seemed to relax as Lady Anne spoke and snorted loudly, between groans, as if in conversation with his owner.

My heart rate dropped by about twenty beats

per minute through sheer relief once I had successfully injected sedative into Trevor's jugular vein. It would take a few minutes before it started to work, which gave me time to quiz Lady Anne about any changes that might have faced Trevor recently — dietary differences, worming procedures, anything that might have brought on this episode. As is often the case with a colicking horse, nothing useful was revealed by my history taking, so there was nothing for it — I would have to start my examination.

The first part of any examination of a horse with colic is to check the pulse and heart rate. We are supposed to feel the pulse under the lower jaw as well as listening to the heartbeat with a stethoscope. They are usually exactly the same, but occasionally the pulse and heart rates are different. Today though, I decided just to listen to his heart, to avoid doing anything around his head that might upset him. Gently, gently, because even in a horse with a very painful belly, the surprise of a cold, metal circular object on the side of its chest can cause alarm.

Trevor's mind, however, was on something else completely and the stethoscope on his side did not bother him one little bit. Now came the time to count. The simple rule is that the faster the heart rate, the more serious the colic. The normal heart rate of a horse is about thirty-two to forty beats per minute. Forty to fifty would fall into the 'mildly elevated' category, fifty to sixty would be 'moderately severe'. Anything over about eighty is in the danger zone, usually signifying extreme pain and carrying a grave prognosis.

I counted the beats up to fifteen seconds on my watch. I repeated it a second and then a third time, just to check, and to make sure the rate was not changing.

'Bother,' I thought.

Trevor's heart rate stubbornly refused to be anything other than fifteen beats in fifteen seconds, which made sixty beats in a minute. That was pretty high and it warranted further investigations, especially since I would have expected his heart rate to have reduced a bit with the sedation. In short, this meant I was going to have to try to palpate Trevor's large intestine, per rectum, and run the risk of being kicked. It is a good idea to lift up one front leg of any horse when this procedure is being undertaken, as it makes it more difficult for them to kick if they have to balance on two legs. As I explained what I needed to do, I knew there was not a chance that Lady Anne could lift up the front leg of this horse.

First, though, I needed to listen to his intestines, to hear what noises were being made. Upper and lower segments, both left and right. I listened patiently. There was a lot of noise, much louder and with much more gurgling than there should have been. Could this simply be a case of spasmodic colic? I really hoped so, because that could be simply treated with a single injection of a spasmolytic. But the horse was in *so much* pain and his heart rate was very high, especially considering that he was sedated. As much as I tried to convince myself that a rectal examination was not necessary, I knew that this was really the correct thing to do.

I could not vacillate for much longer. I watched him intently as I returned from my car with long gloves and lubricant. He looked much more relaxed as a result of the sedative drugs, their painkilling effect and the soothing words of Lady Anne who, despite her diminutive appearance, was proving to be more help than I had expected. Trevor's head hung low and I could see rhythmic breaths blowing from his nostrils against the dew on the short grass. Occasionally he would lift his head and stomp his feet, as another wave of pain gripped his intestines. His ears flicked and his head rose again as soon as he sensed my approach, although I was sure he had no idea of what I was about to inflict upon him.

A rectal examination on a horse sounds like a deadly dangerous thing to perform, but surprisingly most horses tolerate the procedure quite well. The problem is that if something *does* go wrong, and the vet is kicked, it can be a complete disaster. A kick from one or both back legs at such close range would almost certainly leave the vet with at least one broken leg, and possibly a broken arm as well if it isn't withdrawn in time. Being an equine vet is regarded as amongst the most dangerous of professions and recently it was ranked as *the* most dangerous outside the armed forces. The main cause of injury is from a kick from a hind leg. As Trevor danced around when I came close, I did not want to become another statistic.

I explained my plan again to Lady Anne, as I donned the long, green, plastic glove and smothered my hand in lubricant. I slowly edged my way to the action end and lifted Trevor's bushy tail, standing slightly to his left side. If he were to kick out, it would be better if I were standing to one side rather than immediately behind him. His head went up and he whinnied as I started my examination.

'Phew!' was my first thought, and I exhaled loudly. My hand was inside Trevor's rectum and nothing bad had happened so far. Faeces were present and this was a good sign for Trevor. An absence of faeces in the rectum could indicate a blockage further up the bowel and this would be bad. For me, though, it was not so good, because it meant that I had to scoop it all out, one handful at a time, as if I was moving sand on a beach to make the moat around a sand castle. Every time I put my hand back in to remove more, there was the repeated risk of upsetting the colt.

Eventually though I managed to get rid of it all, which allowed me to feel further up to try and find the cause of Trevor's colic. This added yet another degree of risk, because I was more likely to touch a sensitive part of the intestines. Stretched bands of mesentery or distended loops of bowel would be very sore and if I touched them there would be an instant spasm of pain. Furthermore, the deeper in I examined, the harder it became to pull my arm out quickly. Should Trevor twist or drop suddenly, my arm would be broken. It was time for another deep breath. Trevor fidgeted and his front feet danced as I went in past my elbow. There was no pelvic flexure impaction and I could not feel any displaced intestines. As I reached further forwards, towards the nephrosplenic space, Trevor suddenly became very agitated and his head, as well as his front legs started to go upwards. I could see Lady Anne becoming just as anxious, and I pulled out my arm just in time, as Trevor started to spin round, pivoting around the old lady.

Lady Anne let go of the horse as he went down again and started to roll. My examination had obviously upset his painful bowels, but I was fairly confident that there was nothing too serious going on. I got back hold of the lead rope and encouraged him back to his feet. His intestines were still very noisy and his heart rate had gone up to sixty-eight beats per minute.

What should I do next? More tests or should I make a presumptive diagnosis of spasmodic colic?

As I watched Trevor trying to escape from Lady Anne's hold for the umpteenth time, I decided to opt for the latter. I explained that we should give him a spasmolytic injection. This would stop the spasmodic contractions, which were surely the source of his pain.

Trevor realized that the injection meant the end to his ordeal and the minute I stepped away after administering the medication, he jumped in the air and promptly galloped off, still with his head collar and lead rope attached.

'Oh well, never mind,' sighed Lady Anne. 'Let's have a cup of tea.'

I helped the old lady with the kettle, which

was thick with limescale, and I filled up the teapot. It was heavy and I did not want the final part of my visit to end in disaster because of a mishap with boiling water.

I found somewhere to sit amongst the clutter that took up most of the spare space in the living room. The cup of tea tasted pretty terrible, but Lady Anne was clearly feeling happier and it was nice to talk to her and listen to some of the stories about her life. She had been a successful point-to-pointer when she was younger and fitter and the faded pictures on the walls and in frames on the mantelpiece and sideboards showed her in all her former glory.

As the leaves of tea became visible at the bottom of my chipped cup, I knew it was time to bring up the difficult subject of payment. I had been given strict instructions not to leave without a cheque in payment both for today's visit and towards the outstanding balance on the account.

'Lady Anne, would it be possible to have a cheque to pay something off your account, please?' I tried to be as sympathetic as I could.

'Oh dear. I'll see what I can do,' she winced and shuffled across the room towards the bureau in the corner and rummaged inside. When she found the chequebook, it was evident by its size that it was not from a normal, high-street bank. I tried to disguise the widening of my eyes. I had heard about cheques like these, from private banks like Coutts, but I had never seen one before. Suddenly I had less sympathy for the financial plight of the old lady, but Lady Anne went on to explain, as she found a chewed Biro with which to fill out the details of a payment, 'It's very difficult, you see. The rest of my family has all the money. They live on a large estate in Derbyshire, with staff and everything. My sister was really the apple of my mother's eye and she got it all. I haven't really got very much, you know. The stud fees are huge and feed and bedding in the winter is a real burden for me.'

It was so sad. I felt like saying that it was not a problem and that the cheque could wait until another day, but I could imagine how this would go down, back at the practice. I just sat in my chair, shuffling uncomfortably and looking alternately at my feet and the horse pictures on the walls.

It took quite a while for Lady Anne to fill out the cheque. With shaking hands, she handed it over, asking me to complete the 'payee' details on the top line. I realized she hadn't asked me how much she owed. *Thirty pounds* read the spidery writing along the central line of the massive cheque.

'Oh, well. At least I've tried,' I thought, but I knew I would be in trouble. Thirty pounds didn't even cover the cost of the drugs that I had injected into Trevor, let alone the hour or so of veterinary time, fuel costs and so on. It was woefully inadequate, but I didn't feel it was fair to ask for any more. I bade farewell to Lady Anne, promising to visit again later in the day to check that Trevor was responding as I hoped.

I knew it would be difficult to fix up another visit in work time, because I would incur the wrath of Jean in accounts if I added more work to a bill that had an almost zero chance of being paid. So I came up with a cunning plan. The days are long in June in Thirsk and I decided to call back at Sutton Stables after I'd finished work for the day. I needed to take my dog, Paddy, for a walk and it was a perfect opportunity to visit the beautiful lake called Gormire that sits, nestled under the white stone escarpment, surrounded by ancient woodland. The road to Gormire took me right past the field where Trevor had been rolling around and I knew I could check him from the other side of the fence — a safe distance away. As long as I could see that he was grazing happily, I would know he was healthy and that my injections had worked. If he was lying down, as he had been when I first saw him today, it would be a very short or non-existent dog walk that evening and I would have to dice with danger again.

Luckily for me, for Trevor, for my dog and for Lady Anne's chequebook, when I peered over the fence into Trevor's field it appeared that the colt had been completely cured. He was standing with his fellow youngsters, happily nibbling grass and showing no signs of any abdominal pain at all. I could enjoy my evening dog walk in perfect peace. I followed the path to the lake, winding through the beech trees, covered in their vibrant lime-green summer foliage. It was a good way to end another busy, if slightly stressful, day.

Miscellaneous Creatures

Over the last twenty years or so, the range and type of animals that we treat in our mixed practice has changed considerably. Once, our daily routine would involve mostly dairy cows and beef suckler cows and their calves, sheep to lamb and horses with colic. Dogs and cats made up a much smaller percentage of our caseload than they do today. As farming practices have changed, the number of traditional farms with livestock in the area has dwindled, but there has been a significant increase in so-called 'hobby farming'. The mixture of work that we do has correspondingly slowly but surely shifted. It is not uncommon for a round of visits to include a sick goat, an alpaca that has stopped eating or a miniature donkey that needs to be castrated. Even though the commercial imperative of getting a dairy cow back to full milk has largely disappeared from the majority of work in a mixed practice like ours, the role of the veterinary surgeon is just as important, arguably even more so, as people come into farming without prior experience, or branch out into unusual breeds. We treat the pet goat or pet alpaca as exactly that — a pet, a member of the family in just the same way as a rabbit is now considered part of the family, as much as a cat or a dog.

One of our farmers flatly refuses to send her

old 'cull' ewes to market as most other farmers would do, maximizing their profit by selling elderly sheep to the mutton trade. She asks me to visit to euthanase her 'old girls' by injection. She can't bear the idea that they would be sent for meat, after all they have done for her over the years. Many farmers and even some veterinary surgeons would consider this a sentimental approach, but it is not our place to pass judgement.

Some vets shy away from this kind of large animal work — it's not exactly the premier league of vet practice but, to me, it is actually incredibly rewarding. I am asked to the farm to treat the animal because it is sick, not because it has ceased to be productive. It is purely for the animal's benefit and has nothing to do with economics. A keeper of backyard chickens wants her favourite, egg-bound chicken cured, not so that she gets back to her full egg-laying productivity, but because she wants her chicken to be happy and healthy again. To me, it doesn't matter if the patient is a goat, an alpaca, a ferret or a chicken. Any sick animal deserves to have the benefit of veterinary help.

This gradual change in philosophy has certainly been part of the reason for the change in array of our daily patients.

★ ★ ★

The message in the daybook wasn't very helpful. It simply said, '*Julian, please phone Mr Nichols*' and gave his telephone number. This kind of

184

cryptic message always makes for an entertaining phone call. It was around the time when we were in the midst of the Channel 5 series, *The Yorkshire Vet*, and we were getting used to a miscellaneous selection of phone requests. A call might be to congratulate us upon the latest episode, to point out a mistake we'd made on screen ('It was a merlin, *not* a juvenile sparrow hawk!'), or to make a request that I talk at the local WI meeting ('I'd love to, if I can fit it in. How many people will be attending? . . . Oh, about six or eight. Very good, it will be quite informal then? . . . I'll see if I can fit it in. We are quite busy with this sort of thing at the moment').

When I phoned Mr Nichols, he was quick to get to the point.

'Well, I have this donkey. It's a Miniature Mediterranean Donkey. It's got a retained testicle, apparently. My vet says he can't deal with such things. I've seen you lot on the telly and I know that you are the testicle experts. Can I bring it for you to have a look at?'

We do a fair few horse and donkey castrations and they are not so taxing. But the removal of an internal testicle is more complicated altogether. The job usually falls to equine vets who have the facilities to perform a full general anaesthetic and have a fully equipped equine operating theatre. My first thought was that this should be the course of action here and I started to explain this to Mr Nichols. As I was talking, though, I realized that I had never seen a Miniature Mediterranean Donkey. I imagined it would

185

probably be quite small, especially at just six months old, as this one was. I asked about his size.

'Oh, he's about as big as my Labrador, that's all. I can pick him up. I thought I would bring him over to you in my car boot, if that's all right?'

Mr Nichols had thought it all through.

'We live in Beverley, but I don't mind fetching him over.'

This being the case, our small animal operating theatre would be the perfect place to perform the procedure. It would be not very much different to doing the same operation on a Great Dane.

And so we made arrangements for 'Archie' the teenage (in donkey terms) Miniature Mediterranean Donkey to come in. Sure enough, a week later, he was lifted out of the straw-filled boot of Mr Nichols' car, to take his place in the kennels, next to the dogs, cats and rabbits. As he stood in the x-ray room, waiting in the dim light for his sedative to take effect, he was oblivious to the ridiculousness of his situation. Everyone who walked past had to do a double-take when they realized the creature had enormous ears and a head collar instead of a collar and lead.

Everything went very smoothly. Within half an hour, Archie's small but elongated testicles were lying in a metal kidney dish and he was beginning to come round from his anaesthetic. Mr and Mrs Nichols had enjoyed a brief foray into Thirsk for a coffee, but were now back in the waiting room, anxious to take the little man home. Archie could just about totter out to the car park from his kennel (again heads turned) but needed a helping hand into the boot. It had been an unusual morning. Mr and Mrs Nichols were very happy. I think Archie was happy too, but it was hard to tell. His face gave nothing away!

★ ★ ★

The first alpacas to appear around Thirsk in significant numbers came in 2002, the year after the foot and mouth disease outbreak that decimated the nation's cattle and sheep population. Thirsk was badly hit, and many farmers lost all their stock. After this terrible trauma, and after the prescribed time had elapsed before restocking was allowed, farmers turned their thoughts to what to do next. Some saw it as an opportunity to do something new. Ed and Linda, dairy farmers who had lost all their animals in the cull, had taken the opportunity, while they had no twice-daily commitment to the udders of their cows, to enjoy a holiday in South America. It is easy to imagine what happened next. Fields that once were home to over a hundred black and white cows were filled with elegant, long-legged and long-necked creatures whose eyelashes rivalled those of their bovine predecessors and whose fleeces were many times softer than those of the sheep whose fields they adjoined. When visits came through to the practice to see these unusual animals, all the other vets suddenly — or so it seemed — had

187

very important paperwork to do or really urgent dentals to perform, and it was not long before I became the 'alpaca man'.

At this stage I had no specialist knowledge of alpacas. I had established that they were very broadly similar to sheep (although this is a gross oversimplification, as they have numerous subtle and not-so-subtle differences in terms of both the diseases they face and the personality and behaviour they display), but as time went on, I realized that to get to know this type of camelid was to fall in love with them. On my first visit, I found that, quite unlike sheep, which would immediately tend towards fear and flight, these curious animals would come up and investigate whatever was going on. They had no malice and radiated a calm serenity, both in their demeanour and also the gentle noises they made. Standing in a field of alpacas, I discovered, was a calming, tranquil experience.

I was quickly in at the deep end and it was fortunate for me, as well as the herd, that I was fascinated by alpacas, right from the very start. After a handful of missed diagnoses, I started to feel that I knew what I was doing, until one sunny afternoon, when I was called to an alpaca that was struggling to give birth. These animals have enormously long necks and even longer limbs, so if things go wrong at a birth (called by those in the know 'unpacking'), then things go *badly* wrong. My first 'unpacking' was probably one of the most difficult I could have faced. It was a sunny afternoon in the school holidays and my son Jack, who must have been about seven years old, had come with me to work. As I drove onto the farm, I was ushered straight up to the field where the stricken female had been corralled into an outdoor pen. I put on a glove and felt inside to try to establish the cause of her difficulty. I'd done this procedure thousands of times before in sheep, but this was the first time in a camelid.

Jack had a grandstand view from his car seat and as he peered out, my face must have been a picture of confusion as I tried to work out what I was feeling. Then it dawned on me — the alpaca had a uterine torsion. This is a condition where the uterus twists through 180 degrees. The effect it has on the birth canal is the same as that achieved by twisting the top of a bag or the ends of a sweet wrapper — it closes it off completely. The only solution was to perform a caesarian section.

Jack was not the only spectator. Ed, his wife Linda, their son (plus his girlfriend), their daughter and Linda's father, Trevor, were also watching. Trevor was an enthusiast with a hand-held video camera and he had rushed to start filming the action as soon as Ed and Linda had realized there was a problem with the alpaca. He captured every moment. I was used to this, because one of Trevor's first (and my first, for that matter) forays into filming was of me operating on a cow with a twisted stomach. I think he has a large archive of various vets from Skeldale, cutting into all manner of animals on his farm!

With seven onlookers, one with a video

189

camera, the pressure was on, especially as I was in uncharted territory. This was my first 'unpacking' and my first caesarian on an alpaca, but one caesarian is much like another, and I decided to treat the operation as somewhere between a sheep caesarian and the same procedure on a cow, both of which I had performed hundreds of times before. The gentle alpaca remained impeccably behaved throughout and, mercifully, everything went extremely smoothly.

Trevor decided to send his video footage to the local television news, such was the novelty of the event, and a reporter appeared at the surgery to conduct an interview. Linda was so enthusiastic about sharing anything out of the ordinary, and so keen on alpacas, that the next thing I knew there were pictures of me in all the alpaca magazines as well.

By strange coincidence, my second difficult 'unpacking' was also recorded on camera. This time the camera was altogether more fancy and was operated by David, one of the producer-directors of *The Yorkshire Vet*.

On this occasion the practice had received a call from Jackie, who farms a herd of about a hundred breeding alpacas. Jackie is extremely experienced and whenever I get a call from her, I know it is going to be something challenging.

'Julian, it's Cinderella. She's trying to give birth, but I'm really worried that something's wrong. She started in the middle of the night and she's just walking around in the field, with her tail in the air. She's definitely not right.'

This was an emergency. I put all other work

on hold and whizzed out of the car park with David sitting next to me, camera poised to record. As we drove to the farm, David asked questions about what was happening, where we were going and what we might see when we got there. I explained to the camera that alpacas normally give birth with ease and that whenever a problem arises it is usually serious. As we rushed along the winding lanes to Jackie's farm I told David all about the twisted uterus and I could see he was excited — he sensed he was onto a great story to film.

He was not wrong. As I carefully felt inside Cinderella's birth canal, the problem was immediately obvious. All I could feel was a tail. The cria (which is the name for a baby alpaca) was in a breech presentation; that is, it was coming backside first with both back legs pointing forwards, towards the mother's head. This was a very difficult mal-presentation as I would need to manipulate both back legs so they were pointing backwards, towards the way out. In this way I would then be able to deliver the cria, although it would still be coming out backwards rather than forwards. Of all the animals we deal with, alpacas have the longest legs for their body size and this would make the job extremely tricky. There is a real danger, when trying to hook the back legs up and back, that a sharp little hoof will tear the wall of the uterus. In a lamb or calf it is usually possible to cup the hoof in your hand, to protect the delicate tissue, but with such long spindly legs, there was a strong possibility I wouldn't be able to get my hand far enough forwards to do this. Jackie was worried and David honed his focus to capture all the excitement on camera. It could not have been a more tense twenty minutes.

I gave Cinderella an epidural so she would relax from her incessant but unproductive and unhelpful straining. This was critical, as it allowed me to push the cria back a little, giving me space to manipulate the back feet into position. With extreme caution, I managed to turn the feet to where they needed to be, thankfully without inflicting any damage. Finally I could start to pull. At this point it is important to be quick, because once the umbilical cord breaks, the newborn takes its first gasp. This is fine if it is coming forwards, but if it is coming out backwards, it could breathe in a lungful of amniotic fluid rather than air. As I pulled the cria out, back legs first, the enormous length of its limbs became greatly exaggerated, partly because I was pulling quite hard and partly because the slimy mucous covering its entire body slicked down its woolly fleece and made it appear even more lengthy. The baby just kept coming and all I could hear myself saying, rather ridiculously, was, 'Blimey! Look how long it is!'

The cria was a female, and was quickly christened Florence — Jackie already knew what she would call it. She was always prepared, but it was relief that was her overriding emotion as I gathered my kit. She gave Cinderella a hug and then looked at me saying, 'I don't know how you did that, Julian!' I expected a hug too, but it didn't happen. I think I was too slimy!

'Kneepads' the goat was a regular patient and typical of the changing demographic of our large animal patients. His previous owners had sold their farmhouse between Thirsk and Ripon in the summer of 2001 to a couple from London. The solicitors had done their bit and the move was going smoothly. The same could not be said for the workings of the Ministry of Agriculture, Fisheries and Food (MAFF). The countryside was ravaged by foot and mouth disease. Movement restrictions, aimed at reducing the spread of the highly virulent virus around the country, meant that ruminants could only be moved under licence from MAFF. Kneepads could not leave the farm. So, when Hannah and her husband made their move from London to their new house in the country, they also inherited a goat. They didn't really know much about goats.

One Saturday visit read succinctly: '*Visit goat — completely tangled in wire.*' Whilst this was not really a veterinary emergency, the untangling of a goat in the middle of a sunny field with Kneepad's new owners was an entertaining way to spend an hour. And it was by no means the first of such visits. Kneepad's recent clinical notes painted a picture:

Visit goat to trim feet. Unable to catch.
Visit goat: check horns. They are fine.
Visit goat: milk coming out of udder for no apparent reason.
Visit goat: eaten gardening gloves.

These jobs were not particularly technical, but they made for a pleasant (if slightly frustrating) pastime. Luckily, on this occasion, I managed to unravel the goat from the wire without too many problems.

The height of Kneepad's notoriety at Skeldale, however, came the following summer. The naughty goat had broken into the shed where the sheep nuts were kept (Hannah also kept two sheep, to keep the grass down in the paddock and as company for the goat). Kneepads had greedily eaten as much as he could manage and he now had terrible stomachache followed by bad diarrhoea. He was suffering from a condition called ruminal acidosis. This is the result of concentrated food, like sheep nuts, being fermented rapidly in the rumen, and the symptoms can range from being very mild — like indigestion — to very serious or even life-threatening. Hannah phoned the surgery for advice and spoke to Sue. I didn't know what had happened, but I could hear the vet end of the conversation, which went a bit like this.

'I see. That is a very greedy goat, then. He sounds like he has developed something called ruminal acidosis. Have you got any bicarbonate of soda in your kitchen cupboard?'

I knew exactly what Sue had in mind, but I also knew that Hannah would be baffled. Was baking the solution to Kneepads' tummy ache? Did he need cake? Luckily, Sue was quick to explain. The plan was not to make buns for Kneepads, but to mix a tonic for the goat, using the bicarbonate of soda. This alkaline solution would then counteract the acidity in the rumen, caused by the excessive fermentation of the sheep food. Sue continued to give clear instructions.

'Right, that's good.' There had obviously been a positive response to the request for bicarb. 'You need to mix about two teaspoons with water in an empty wine bottle. Shake it up until it has dissolved and then use it to drench the goat.'

There was clearly a surprised silence at the other end of the phone.

Sue continued, as she rolled her eyes, 'Trust me. It's what you need to do. It will help. I'm just about to start evening surgery, but give me a ring in an hour or so if he's no better and I can come and have a look. It's easy to do, but drench him now. It's sure to help. You can't go wrong. As long as you pour it nice and slowly.'

Sure enough, when evening surgery had finished and a few of us were getting ready to go for a quick pint in our favourite pub, the Blacksmith's Arms, Sue was heading out to see the goat.

'I'm off to see this blooming goat. It's got acidosis and the owners haven't got a clue. They've asked me to go out — it's no better.'

'Never mind, Sue,' I commiserated. 'Call in at the Blacksmith's after you're done. We're off for a quick drink. We'll be sitting out the back — it's a lovely evening for it. I'll get you a gin — you look like you'll need it!'

Forty-five minutes later, Sue appeared in the beer garden with a massive grin all over her face and an amusing story to tell.

'The goat lady met me as I got out of my car and I could tell she wasn't very happy. She said, 'I've done as you said, but it has made absolutely no difference. Come and have a look.' So I followed her around the corner and into the shed. The goat was standing there, looking at me with his head on one side. His abdomen was still bloated and he was soaking wet! She'd poured the whole mixture all over him! He looked quite confused and his ears were drooping. I shouldn't have, but I just burst out laughing there and then!'

Sue had failed to explain that 'drenching' a goat (or any other farm animal, for that matter) is the process of tipping the mixture, remedy or tonic down its throat, rather than drenching it in the manner one would become drenched by standing out in the rain. No wonder Kneepads was not feeling better after his drenching — it was more of a soaking! Hannah had learnt another lesson in farming, and Sue had realized that some of our newer large animal customers needed more guidance than others.

The Great Yorkshire Show

The summer of 2015 was proving to be one full of hurdles for Martin and his herd of Dairy Shorthorn cattle. He had all his hopes pinned on 'Empress', his best cow, to win 'Best in Class' in the Junior Cow category at the Great Yorkshire Show. He had shown her to me proudly earlier in the year, when I had visited to scan some of his heifers for pregnancy.

He explained how critical her calving date was in relation to the timing of the show.

'If she calves at just the right time, she'll have the right amount of nature in her bag. It's all about the nature, you see. If it comes right, she's got a chance of winning.'

I had never heard the term 'nature' in this context before, but I assumed it described the amount of filling or swelling of the udder. He went on, 'So, Julian, what you tell me with your scanner today is of critical importance to me.'

Martin was almost hopping from foot to foot as he ushered the heifers into position, so I could scan each one in turn. I worked my way down the byre, ticking each one off as I checked it for pregnancy. They were all pregnant. Finally, it was the turn of Empress, a lovely-looking golden brown and white cow, fastened up by halter at the end of the row.

I had encountered Empress for the first time shortly after the Great Yorkshire Show a year earlier. Martin's hopes for her were dashed when the veterinary surgeon on duty at the show diagnosed that she was suffering from a displaced abomasum. This is a condition whereby the fourth chamber of the stomach floats up into the wrong position and becomes trapped between the rumen and the body wall. It can go unnoticed for a while, but eventually causes the cow to go off her food and lose condition. Empress wasn't particularly poorly, but Martin was forced to take her home without so much as setting foot in the show ring. He called me in straight away to operate to correct the problem. The procedure went smoothly. I repositioned her displaced stomach back where it was supposed to be, in the lower right-hand part of her abdomen, and stitched it securely in place. Before long, she was eating and ruminating normally and — critically for her chances in the show ring — her wounds had healed up perfectly, with no trace of a scar.

Martin could hardly watch while I carried out Empress's pregnancy test. I inserted my lubricated probe, found the uterus and peered at the image on the screen of the scanner.

'Good news, Martin!' I announced. 'She's in calf and about ten weeks. That means she should calve at the end of June.'

As I looked up from the screen, I could see Martin jumping up and down with excitement and delight. He punched the air and high-fived Vladik, his Latvian assistant. It is normal for farmers to be pleased to hear the news that a cow is pregnant, but Martin's excitement was on another level. Vladik was a loyal helper, but often struggled to understand exactly what Martin was saying and I was not convinced that he knew the reason for Martin's ecstatic joy.

Once he had stopped jumping up and down, Martin confirmed that this calving date meant that Empress's perfect udder would be at just the right tightness (or 'nature', as Martin referred to it) to impress the judges at Harrogate. It would put her at a significant advantage in the ring. The odds of winning were now stacked in her favour, provided she stayed healthy, calved without any problems and reached peak condition in time for the important date at the beginning of July. It was Martin's dream to follow in his uncle's footsteps and win the title of Dairy Shorthorn Champion at the Great Yorkshire Show. It had taken him nearly twenty years to get to this point and he sensed that the fulfilment of his dream was now within his grasp.

Needless to say, I visited Empress many times throughout the rest of the year, keeping a close eye on her health, in the run-up to the prestigious show. She calved uneventfully, although Martin had many sleepless nights, constantly checking to ensure she was not in trouble. Four days after she had calved, though, I received a frantic telephone call.

'Julian, I'm worried. It's Empress. She's not cleansed,' said Martin. After calving, Empress had not passed the afterbirth. This can lead to serious illness and Martin knew this all too well. 'Now she's gone right off her cake. Her milk's dropping right off too. Can you come and have a look? I'm worried she has got another twisted stomach. Can you come now?'

I tried to reassure him. 'I'll be right there, Martin. Don't worry. I'm sure we can sort her out.'

I could hear the worry in his voice but I knew that it was very unlikely that her stomach had displaced again. I had sutured it in position securely and I was sure it could not have come undone. I'd never known this happen before and I had done the procedure many times.

Martin met me halfway down the drive of the farm and talked constantly as we walked into the dark byre where Empress was penned with her calf. I could see immediately that she was not well. Her eyes were dull and her sides were hollow rather than showing the healthy round-ness that accompanies a full rumen.

'Can we get her in the crush, Martin?' I asked.

'Of course we can.' Martin sprang into action. 'Vladik, Vladik! Come here! Help me get Empress into the crush! Come on, Vladik, let's get a move on. You push and I'll pull!'

Within minutes, Empress found herself standing in the cattle crush, the same one that she had been standing in nearly a year ago as I rummaged around her insides. We all hoped I would not need to do the same today, as this would put an end to her chances of becoming a champion.

Luckily for Empress and for Martin, the abomasum was exactly where it should have been (and exactly where I left it). There was not a trace of the telltale 'pinging' sound that all

200

large animals vets know so well, and is a sure sign of a displaced stomach. We all (including Vladik, even though he still didn't really know what was going on) breathed a sigh of relief. I checked her temperature. It was high but not dangerously so. Then I felt inside her vagina with my gloved hand. Sure enough, her cleansing — the remains of the placenta, which had attached her calf to the inside of her womb during pregnancy — was still partially attached. It was smelly and beginning to decompose. This was the cause of her ill health and needed to be removed. With a gentle pull, it slid out easily and I placed a handful of antibiotic pessaries inside, to treat the infection. A couple of injections later and with the rotting membranes on the floor of the barn rather than sitting inside her uterus, I was confident that Empress would be fine. Martin was relieved, but I knew that, even with the enhanced feeding regime that would now be put in place, his hopes of winning the top prize had been severely dented. The show was only two weeks away. His beloved cow would be safe, which was the most important thing to him, but would she pick up enough condition and would her udder recover the required 'nature' to clinch the red rosette? Only time would tell.

As I left the farm, I promised Martin I would be at the ringside to see Empress in all her glory in two weeks' time at the Great Yorkshire Show, but as a spectator rather than a vet.

Two weeks later, even in the middle of a heaving Harrogate show ground, Martin was not difficult to find. I followed the signs to the area designated for dairy cattle. Normally, my first instinct would have been to head straight to the beef section. I always think that beef cattle are much more handsome and impressive to look at than the skinny, catwalk types of dairy cow, which often give the impression that they would be blown over by a strong gust of wind. I skirted past these dainty black and white size zeros and, when I found the Dairy Shorthorn area, there was no missing Martin and his entourage. Deck chairs had been arranged in a long phalanx down the middle of the building for all of Martin's friends and helpers. Wendy, the cow beautician from West Yorkshire, had been busy during the small hours and Empress looked a picture. Her hair was neatly trimmed, her topline was immaculate and her udder looked full of nature. I could see, though, that despite the extra food she had been given over the last fortnight her recent illness had taken its toll — the bones on her back and around her tail-head protruded just a hint more than they should. But, despite this, Martin was standing next to her like a proud father.

I negotiated my way around the other groups of farmers, still trimming and brushing their cows, and made my way over to Martin and his group. He was fastidiously fluffing up Empress's tail using a special tool for the job.

'Morning, Martin. How are you feeling today?'

'To tell you the truth, Julian, I'm nervous. Confident but nervous.' Martin's tone told me exactly how anxious he was. 'She looks well, and she's healthy and happy, her bag's full of nature

— but whether she'll win, Julian, who knows? We've done our best, but once we go into that ring, it's down to the judges.'

Martin turned back to Empress, and threw up his hands in horror.

'Oh, shit! Vladik, pass me that paper towel. Empress has crapped all down herself!'

The immaculate cow had raised her tail and relieved her bowels, yet again. Maybe she was feeling the nerves, too?

Vladik put down the broom that he had been using to tidy up the straw in the cow's bed, and came to help clean the cow's bottom. Vladik's sister, Veronika, had also come along to give moral support, and she sat on one of the deck chairs, eating an ice cream. Her filmstar good looks were partly hidden by an enormous pair of round, black sunglasses and it was an incongruous sight — the juxtaposed images of a model on a fashionable beach in the South of France mixed with a holidaymaker on Scarborough seafront, with the donkey that might have been standing by having been replaced by an immaculately presented Dairy Shorthorn!

I had met Veronika before, when I had treated her cat Lucy, who had been suffering from a severe form of cancer. Veronika was emotionally traumatised by Lucy's illness, not only because of her devotion to her pet, but also because she believed that a pet's illness foretold of similar misfortunes that were in store for its owner. It had been a difficult time. I went over to talk to her, hoping that I would not rekindle sad memories of her cat.

'Good morning, Veronika. Empress looks very well today. Fingers crossed!' I offered.

'Empress very pretty cow. They all very pretty cow,' she replied in her flat, heavy Latvian accent, between licks of her ice cream.

'Yes, you are right. They are all very pretty cows.' And with this I knew our conversation had come to an end.

I said goodbye to Martin and his gang, wishing him the very best of luck before heading off to explore the show. I made sure I was back in time to watch the class being judged.

I know quite a lot about cows, but I am always flummoxed by the criteria used by the judges, as they stare silently from under their bowler hats at the magnificent cattle processing round and round the show ring. Today, I knew that the preference of the judge would make or break my friend. I also suspected that Martin had secretly resigned himself to the fact that any rosette would be a victory, under the circumstances of Empress's recent illness.

The man on the loudspeaker announced the results as the judge made his decisions, calling out the number of each cow. The number was also emblazoned on the front of each handler, like an enormous version of the number an athlete would wear in a race. First and second were announced in order and, watching from the side, I willed the third number to match the one on Martin's chest.

'And the prize for third place in this class goes to number one-one-four-seven,' announced the commentator.

Martin's face briefly lit up as he glanced down to his chest to check his number. I could see clearly that it didn't match. Martin's number was one-one-four-six. My heart sank. I knew he would be disappointed.

Later on, after the cows had been put back in their stalls and the excitement of the day had passed, I called back to see Martin. He was slumped in one of the deck chairs with a can of caffeinated soft drink balanced in the cup holder. He was fast asleep. It had been a long few days for him and his team and he was exhausted. Maybe next year would be his year.

Thunderbolts and Lightning

The weather in summer in the Vale of York, the Hambleton and Howardian Hills and the North York Moors is not always gloriously sunny. On occasions we have our very own version of the monsoon. After days of nonstop heat, scorching the crops and bleaching the grass, the humidity always rises. Storm clouds gather over just a few hours and the culmination is a series of electrical storms, often of biblical proportions. Because cattle are always out grazing at this time of year and because they tend to group themselves together, seeking shelter under trees or, for some unfathomable reason, hanging around near electricity pylons, they seem to act as excellent lightning conductors. Standing in wet mud, as they do, a group of about twenty animals each weighing about 500 kilograms and made up, basically, of salty electrolytes seems to attract lightning very readily, as the electric discharge seeks the path of least resistance to earth.

My first experience of this was one Saturday afternoon, soon after I graduated. There was a call to a beef farm to see a group of adult cattle, in the midst of a terrible storm. I was at the surgery, locking the doors having attended to a sick dog. Rain lashed down on the windows and roof, and water cascaded over the gutters and spouted out of the drains. It lasted no more than ten or fifteen minutes, but before the torrential rain had stopped, my beeper went off.

The farmer was in a terrible state and through the roar of the rain at both his end of the phone and mine, I could barely make out what he was saying. I assured him that I was on my way and would be with him very soon. At least I would be once I had found my way to the car, across what should have been the car park but was now a lake.

The rain eased before too long, which was just as well because the windscreen wipers on my trusty old Ford Escort would not have coped with the volume of water that had been hurling out of the sky. I trundled along the dual carriageway, not wanting to get up too much speed in all the spray, before turning off down the farm track. The farmer was standing with his young son halfway down the lane and they waved me into a gateway, some distance from the farm itself. My car was steamed up and I couldn't see the macabre spectacle in the field. As I wound down the window, both father and son started to talk at once.

'We have eleven cattle, all dead. They were standing near this metal gate and, well, Andy, you tell the vet what happened,' garbled the farmer before deferring to his son, who seemed years ahead of his teenage looks.

'I couldn't believe it, Vet'nary. I was out on my bike and suddenly it started tipping down with rain — proper heavy, it was. I stopped halfway down that hill and sheltered under a tree, just to get out of the rain, really, and suddenly there was a massive bang. Then, the rain eased off where I was and I came down here to this field. Next to this metal gate — just here — all these young heifers were just lying here, all dead, their legs sticking out and all lined up next to each other. They must have toppled over, just like dominoes. Some were twitching but they must have been dead 'cos smoke was coming from them all. I couldn't believe my eyes, so I set off back up the hill and got me dad to phone you up. I think they must have been struck by lightning!'

The young lad was right. As I got out of the car it was evident that my veterinary skills were redundant. Nearly a dozen strong, fully grown cattle lay side by side, just like toppled dominoes. Smoke was, indeed, still rising from some of them. It was a sight that I would never forget. The cattle must have been standing with their noses pressed up to the metal gate when it was hit with a deafening crash by the bolt of lightning. The enormous voltage had surged to earth by the route of least resistance and all the animals were dead.

The smell was as disturbing as the sight, as the aroma of a vigorous barbecue — typical of those stoked up by barbecue diehards who stubbornly persist with al fresco cooking, even though the weather is rubbish — hung in the wet air.

There was nothing I could do, other than to certify that the animals were dead, so that the farmer could claim on his insurance. I took down their ear tag numbers and (as it was before the era of the smart phone) took some photos with the little camera I carried in my glove box to document the tragedy. It must have been an instantaneous death for the poor animals, but this was of little comfort as the three of us gawped, shocked and useless.

It was utterly bad luck and a freak accident. Nothing could have been done to prevent it.

There was another farm, not far from the site of this tragedy, to which we would be called after almost any electrical storm. Yet another bovine would be lying dead, close to a pylon or electricity pole and our role was to examine the carcass and pronounce upon whether or not it had been struck by lightning. The call would always come in a day or so after the storm, so any smoke would have long since subsided. In fact, there were almost never any specific signs of a lightning strike and it was very difficult to confirm the exact cause of death. Crucially, most insurance policies cover sudden death by lightning strike. The farmer would throw up his hands and say casually, 'Oh, can you just put down that it's dead? The insurance people don't mind. Just as long as there is a vet certificate.'

So I would write a letter, stating that I had examined a heifer that had been found dead the morning after an electrical storm, that I could find no obvious cause of death, that it *may* have been killed by a lightning strike, but that I could not confirm this. It was true and I would have been happy to have discussed the vagueness of my diagnosis with anybody, but this never seemed to be necessary.

'Oh, that'll be fine. I'll give it to the insurance, thank you,' I would be assured.

It always was, and nobody from the insurance

company ever contacted me for more information, but I feel sure they must have smelt a rat!

★ ★ ★

It was another weekend in the middle of summer, and another thunderstorm was threatening, when my Sunday lunch was rudely interrupted by the insistent beeping of my pager. One of Gordon's Dexter cows was calving and it was not progressing as it should. Gordon was a very experienced farmer and calls to his herd of short and stocky Dexter cattle were always tough. I knew I would not be enjoying my pudding for some time.

Dexters are a miniature breed of cattle, originating from Ireland. Their small size meant they were perfect to provide milk for a single family, without needing as much forage and space as one of their larger cousins. They were bred from mountain cattle and I am sure these hardy origins must be part of the reason why these cattle are so stubborn. For all that they are just half the size of a standard breed, they are often at least twice as difficult to handle, and stubbornly refuse to cooperate or to be herded into the appropriate places. This was exactly the case today. The pregnant cow was standing resolutely in the far distance. Gordon and his son, Toby, pointed out the tiny black speck about a quarter of a mile away, and filled me in on the details. She had been calving for a couple of hours. The water bag had burst before lunchtime.

'And no, we can't get her to move,' finished Gordon resignedly, as he pre-empted my next question. 'We'll have to go to her, I'm afraid,' he apologized, as he offered to fill up my bucket with water.

Luckily, the field in which she was planted was flat, dry and had short grass, so it was an easy job to drive to her, through a couple of gates. I only spilt half of the bucket of water that I had placed in the footwell of my passenger seat, as I followed Gordon and Toby, trundling slowly along in their tractor. At least with half the water still in the bucket, I felt the first part of the challenge had been completed with some success. Judging by the intense blackness of the approaching storm clouds, lack of water was unlikely to be high up on our list of problems.

Most of Gordon's cattle were used to the show ring. They were regular winners at the Great Yorkshire Show, the Royal Highland Show and the Royal Welsh (in fact, Gordon and Toby had returned from a show just the previous day, with another armful of rosettes). This meant that even the most stubborn of his Dexters, who wouldn't be rounded up, and most certainly wouldn't go into a crush, would easily and readily take a halter. So, instead of chasing the cow around the six-acre field for an hour, which is often what happens when trying to catch a Dexter, we could quickly and efficiently attach her to the back of Gordon's tractor by means of a strong rope halter.

'Have you had a feel inside?' I asked Gordon. Usually he would have done so, and made his own assessment of the situation.

'Naw. We've not had time. We've only just got back from feeding the other show cattle. I had a look at her this morning, but as she wasn't getting on wi' it, we thought it was a job for you.'

I lubed up my right arm and cautiously felt inside the short-legged cow. It didn't take long to work out the cause of the problem. The feet of the calf were massive and the head was not engaging. There was no doubt that it was too big to be born naturally. I explained my findings to Gordon and Toby, who didn't need any persuading — in fact they almost handed me the scalpel.

'Whatever you do, you'd better be quick, else we're all gonna get soaked!'

We all looked up to the rapidly approaching storm. It was half an hour away, I reckoned, maybe less. If it arrived before the al fresco operation was finished, it would spell disaster. The three of us getting soaked was the least of our worries. Water running down the cow's back was sure to result in serious wound contamination, and this would make post-operative complications a certainty. If the rain was accompanied by thunder and lightning we would be extremely vulnerable. The metal tractor, the cow and I were all very closely connected and we were the only structures around. We would make a perfect lightning conductor. With my arms elbow-deep in the cow, it would not just be Dexter smoke that would rise skywards.

I had to be quick.

'Hey, Dad. Let's get that gazebo,' suggested

Toby. 'The one we used yesterday at the show. It'll cover the vet and this cow nicely. It's still in one piece — I put it up last night outside the house so I could give it a good clean.'

It was an excellent plan, but since the cow was attached to the tractor, Gordon and Toby had to go back to the farm on foot to fetch the gazebo. As I prepared for the caesarian, clipping hair, injecting the local and scrubbing the left flank, I glanced alternately between the two figures fading into the distance, and the impending storm. By the time father and son had reached the gate at the edge of the field, I had made my incision and was feeling for the calf inside the cow's abdomen. Luckily I had put on my head-torch before starting the operation, because even though it was the early part of a July afternoon, the sun had been completely obliterated by the thick black storm clouds, and it was just like a solar eclipse. I estimated I had about fifteen minutes before we would need an ark, rather than a gazebo.

'Maybe Gordon and Toby should abandon their gazebo mission and start gathering animals, two by two,' I joked with the cow. She didn't appreciate my humour.

As surgeons, we are taught to be quick and efficient. This is important. The longer an animal's abdomen is open, the bigger the risk of infection because, however sterile the environment, the greater the chance of bacteria and other debris entering the body cavity. Keeping surgery short is the key to success. This is especially so when operating in fields or in

213

stables or barns, where sterility of the environment cannot be guaranteed. Today, with black clouds, flashes and rumbles of thunder rapidly getting closer, I needed speed and efficiency more than ever. I reached in and found the calf's hock inside the uterus. I made a curved incision through the uterine wall, over the hock and as far as the foot. Through this opening, I could manipulate the second foot into place and the calf was soon out, landing with a 'plop' on the lush, green grass, that with the pending deluge would shortly be many times more green and lush. The calf spluttered and flapped its ears, peering around. It was happily oblivious to everything.

My next step was to repair the incisions I had made into the uterus, muscle layers and skin. As I reached over for my sutures, I could just see, in the far distance, the meandering progress of a fully erected gazebo, zigzagging from side to side, through the apple trees in the small orchard outside the farmhouse. I felt I should rename the pair 'Paul and Barry' as I could just imagine them shouting 'To me! To you!' at each other, just like the Chuckle Brothers. Their progress was painfully slow and, crucially, much slower than the progress of the black clouds. They had made it through the trees by the time I had closed the uterus. I just had muscle and skin left to go, but raindrops were beginning to spot down here and there, and the wind had started to swirl, causing the newborn and still wet calf to shiver.

I closed the muscle in two swift and continuous layers and moved quickly onto the skin, willing the downpour to hold off for just a few more minutes. Paul and Barry (as they were now called, in my mind) were still a hundred metres away and had clearly abandoned their attempt to reach the cow and me. They had set down their canopy and were both standing huddled underneath it, in anticipation of the full onslaught of the weather.

I placed the final suture, sprayed the wound with blue spray and gave the cow her injections of painkiller and precautionary antibiotic, just as large and heavy raindrops started to pelt me with such force that they were painful on my exposed skin. I quickly untied the cow from the tractor, whipped off the halter and jumped into the car, still plastered in blood and goo from the op, as the heavens opened. The new mother licked her baby, unperturbed by the storm. It was the calf that I felt sorry for. It had only been in the world for twenty minutes — it must have thought that life was like this every day!

Students

During the summer, students descend upon veterinary practices all over the country. Veterinary students spend term time studying the academic stuff but during the university holidays, when those studying other subjects can get a job or go travelling, vet students are required to 'see practice' in veterinary clinics, where they can learn important clinical skills and start to practise some of what they have been taught at vet school.

Once the summer holidays start, practices like Skeldale are full of students, keen to learn. They want to ask lots of questions, take lots of blood samples, interpret as many x-rays as they can, palpate lots of cows' ovaries and do some minor surgical procedures. Of course, all of this is under the close supervision of the veterinary surgeons and is the very best way to learn the practical side of the job. Much of the responsibility for training students in the actual hands-on skills required to become a competent vet is placed upon practitioners. There simply are not sufficient cases at the vet schools of the normal day-to-day type that we deal with all the time in practice. There are plenty of complicated conditions and highly technical surgeries, referred to the specialist teams, but while these are fascinating, they are not the things a new graduate will be dealing with in their first days and weeks of work.

There is no formal arrangement between the universities and veterinary surgeons in practice. There is just the long-standing, unwritten agreement that we will help. We were all students once, and it is good for everyone if budding veterinary surgeons get plenty of practice and support.

For our part, though, it can sometimes be tricky. Our main priority is always to our patients and their owners. It is not fair to use them as 'guinea pigs' on which students can practise. However, if we can get the right balance, and if our students are keen, pleasant and competent, it is very nice to have them 'seeing practice' with us. It's great to share knowledge and sometimes it can be useful to have another pair of hands. We have had a fair selection of interesting students over the years and Tom was one of the most memorable.

When I cycled past the practice on my way back from a Sunday evening cycle ride, I spotted a square, dark green military vehicle parked in the field opposite. I slowed down to have a closer look. We didn't see many vehicles like this in Thirsk. At this time I didn't know that it belonged to Tom, the student who would be with us for the next two weeks.

The following morning, when I drove into work, I noticed that the vehicle was still in the field. The next thing I spotted was the smiling face of our latest student, as he appeared from the kennels. He was being shown round the practice by the head nurse.

He thrust out a hand to introduce himself. 'Hi! I'm Tom. I'm seeing practice with you for the next two weeks. I'm keen to learn what I can, so give me a shout if you have any interesting calls to do. I'm staying nearby so I can come out with you on night-time visits too, if that's okay? Here's my mobile number,' and he scribbled a number on a bit of paper and handed it over.

'Very good. It's nice to see someone keen!' I nodded. 'Where are you staying?' I could tell by his accent that he wasn't local.

'Well, at the moment I'm staying just there.' He pointed over the road to the place where I had seen the unusual olive-coloured vehicle. 'But I'll need to move. I don't think the farmer is very happy that I've camped up in his field. He's already been round to tell me to move. He calmed down a bit when I explained I was coming to work with you lot at the vets, but I need to find somewhere else to put it before the end of the day.'

It all made sense now! The enterprising Tom had solved the problem of finding somewhere to stay on a student budget by converting the old army vehicle into some sort of camper van. Usually, the first thing students do when they arrive to see practice is learn how to castrate a cat, while also trying to commit to memory the names of all the practice staff. However, Tom's first job was to find somewhere to park for the next fortnight. I thought I knew who would be able to help. After I'd finished morning surgery, I made a phone call to Jeanie Green.

'Morning, Jean! How are you today?'

'Not so bad today, Julian. How's your sweet supply?'

Jeanie always kept us supplied with chocolates and boiled sweets and would bring in a consignment on a weekly basis, or whenever she perceived our energy levels might be dropping.

'It's pretty good at the moment, Jeanie, thank you. I wanted to ask if you could help? We have a student here for a couple of weeks. He's called Tom and he is looking for a nearby farm where he can put his camper van. He's a nice lad but he can't keep it in the field opposite the practice. He just needs some water and a space and he'll pay you. Do you think he could come to you?'

'That's fine,' said Jeanie, without a second thought. 'Send him round. No need for any money. I'd be happy to help, lad.'

And so a special relationship developed.

Later that day, Tom's large, box-shaped military vehicle rumbled along behind me, down Long Street and to one of the fields on Jeanie Green's farm. Jeanie came hobbling out of her farmhouse waving her hand above her head, partly to greet us and partly to direct Tom's mobile home to the correct part of the farm. He pulled in through the green metal gates at the far end of the farm buildings, past the Dutch barn, the elderly grey tractor and various other bits of farm machinery, and into the field with the cows.

'That's it. You'll be right in there!' shouted Jeanie, as she signalled Tom into position near the hawthorn hedge. Tom jumped down from his cockpit, leaping over the three steps that led up to the door, and bounded over to introduce himself again, this time to the quirky farmer. The truck was an incredible-looking vehicle and I

219

couldn't wait to peer inside, but Jeanie was quite used to strange things and was completely unfazed by it. I was left to scrutinize it myself as the two went off to find the water supply. A few minutes later, Jeanie emerged from the farm-house wielding three ice creams.

'There you go, lad! Have one of these!'

We all sat around on bales of hay and tucked in. Tom told us about his peculiar method of transport and its provenance.

It was an ex-Russian troop carrier that he had converted into a very basic camper van. Tom explained how, amazingly, it could run on either petrol or diesel, or a combination of the two. He could run it very cheaply by calling at filling stations and collecting the mixture of petrol and diesel that had been drained from the tanks of cars whose drivers had inadvertently filled up with the wrong type of fuel. This seemed unlikely to me, but Tom assured me that this was really the case.

Tom turned out to be just as enthusiastic with his veterinary studies as he was with his mechanical ingenuity, and started to hone some excellent veterinary skills during his stay. He fitted in perfectly at our practice and also with the Greens. He ate tea with them every evening, manfully filling his belly with the hefty meat and potato pies that were Jeanie's speciality. After his allotted two weeks, Tom had put on about a stone in weight, thanks to Jeanie's generous hospitality. He said goodbye, never to be seen again. It was sad, because he was a dynamic and interesting character, and I would have loved to have offered him a job, once he had qualified.

Just as quirky and just as interesting, but possibly less suited to a job at Skeldale, was Angus. He was with us during a spectacularly hot period of weather, the likes of which make it a struggle to cope in the waterproof outfits that we have to wear, to protect our clothes from the dirty environment of a farm. The feeling of sweat trickling down the inside of your trousers is a uniquely unpleasant one. I was seriously considering wearing my shorts, even though I knew it would incur the wrath of my senior colleague. (Not to wear a tie was considered unprofessional behaviour, so the exposure of one's knees and ankles would surely demand an appointment with the Disciplinary Committee of the Royal College of Veterinary Surgeons!)

I had a call to see a bull suffering from heatstroke. I thought it would be an interesting case for a student, so I went to find Angus. I had not seen much of him during the time he had been with us, and this was the first time he had accompanied me. Heatstroke is an unusual condition to affect a farm animal — it is typically seen in dogs if they have been left in a hot car or have been chasing a ball or a frisbee to excess on a hot day. On this occasion, though, it was a one-tonne stock bull that had succumbed. He had been happily mating with cows, oblivious to the blazing midday sun. His vigour had caused him to overheat.

Angus was lurking in the far end of the operating theatre, apparently engrossed in the detail of the inner workings of a cat.

221

'Come on, Angus, we have an interesting case to see. You'll not see many cases of heatstroke in cattle. I'll meet you in the car park.'

He didn't exactly jump at the chance to see this unusual case, but I hadn't really given him the option to decline my offer. It was some time before he emerged from the side door of the practice, carrying a large bag of equipment — wellies, overalls and so on — which he dumped on the back seat of the car.

On the way to the farm, as I always did with students, I quizzed him on the possible differential diagnoses for a recumbent bull (that is, the list of all the possible causes). Angus was short on ideas for what conditions, other than heatstroke, we would need to consider. He was also short on ideas for what we should do when we got there. I guessed that this was not something he had been taught at vet school, although I also knew that veterinary students were taught to apply basic principles to every case, so that if they came across something they hadn't seen before, they could work it out from these principles.

The twenty-minute journey seemed to last forever. Retrieving any ideas from Angus was like pulling teeth. Eventually, we arrived at the farm and drove into the farmyard. Malcolm, the worried farmer, showed me where to go and I bounced through the field as far as I could, before leaving the car on the near side of a hedge. The bull was lying on its side in the next field and I could just make out its enormous bulk. I jumped out and grabbed my thermometer. This was obviously the first step of the examination — even Angus had

222

worked that one out. As I inserted the thermometer and waited for the mercury to rise, I realized that Angus had not followed me through the hedge. Worried that something was wrong, I asked Malcolm, who had followed us across the field in his tractor, to go back and check that he hadn't headed in the wrong direction and got lost.

Moments later Malcolm reappeared through the hole in the hedge, hardly able to speak he was laughing so hard.

'Your mate is just coming,' he just about managed to splutter between gales of laughter. 'He's still getting dressed!'

After I had checked and rechecked the thermometer reading — it was 106°F, way hotter than normal — Angus eventually appeared. He was dressed from head to foot in protective clothing, not just of the type to keep farmyard muck off, but also sufficient to prevent the ingress of a single ray of sunshine. He was wearing wellies and waterproof trousers (standard) but also a long, white smock which extended right to his feet and covered his arms all the way to his hands. On his head was a French Foreign Legion-type hat, with a large peak at the front and an overhanging flap at the back to protect his neck. His nose was smothered with a thick layer of zinc oxide paste. He looked as if he was preparing for a trek across the desert, rather than a fifteen-minute examination of a hot bull in North Yorkshire. Trying not to laugh at this ridiculous sight I glanced up at Malcolm who was, by now, bent double with mirth.

'Wow, Angus, that's some outfit! I've not seen many students dressed up like that before. Are you okay?'

'Yes, thank you, I'm fine,' he replied, rather defensively, from under his hat. 'I just don't like taking chances. The sun can be very strong in summer.'

'Aye lad, it can, but not that strong. Not in North Yorkshire anyway,' gasped Malcolm, before he fell about laughing again.

After several buckets of water from the nearby stream, the bull started to cool down, and recovered uneventfully. Sadly, the same could not be said for the reputation of our budding veterinarian and Malcolm could never keep a straight face when I brought a student with me to his farm forever after.

AUTUMN

Summer always slips slowly and seamlessly into autumn. Other seasons can crash against one another, with a late snowstorm in the middle of May or a seductively mild spell during February, but the month of September is always benign and gentle. If there is such a thing as a quiet time in a mixed practice, it is in early autumn. The cattle are still outside, enjoying the last of the grass, and the lambs have grown and are ready for market.

There are, however, some weird veterinary conditions that appear only in autumn — odd diseases that do not occur at any other time of year, and have you scratching your head, until you remember, 'Ah yes, autumn.' Rye grass staggers is the best example. It is a rare and peculiar neurological disease, which causes grazing cattle to run backwards — actually backwards. Harvest mites, those tiny orange and intensely itchy clusters found between dogs' toes or on cats' ears, are only ever seen at the end of August, and 'fog fever', a toxic type of pneumonia, only occurs in autumn when cattle are turned out onto the last flush of grass before winter.

Many of the farms around Thirsk grow cereals, mainly wheat and barley, which turn golden through the summer, and are harvested in the autumn. Much of this is then used to feed cattle. These cattle have been born and reared on the uplands of Northumberland or Scotland and then sold as 'stores' at the cattle markets in Hexham, Wooler or Bentham. It is common for farmers to buy a hundred head of these store cattle and feed them, lavishly and lovingly, on the barley that they have grown over the summer. It is a simple system and it works well, but is fraught with the risk of pneumonia. The young cattle are moved to new and unfamiliar surroundings, brought indoors and possibly also mixed with animals that have come from other farms, all at the time when the temperature is dropping and the damp autumn mists are descending on the Vale of York. This is the perfect cocktail for respiratory disease, so as autumn progresses, we are kept busy, injecting cattle to save their precious and delicate lungs from the ravaging effects of pneumonia.

But still, it is a beautiful time of year and my favourite time of year. A quiet tranquility settles over the countryside, as all its growing and flowering and producing is done for another year.

Sheep and Simmentals by the River Swale

I hadn't had a very good week. Monday and Tuesday had seen me blood testing a flock of six hundred sheep to check them for a viral infection called Maedi Visna. The flock had been accredited free of this disease, but the last routine flock test had flagged up two positive cases. This was disastrous. They had lost their accreditation. As the animals were a high quality, high pedigree flock, it was crucial to be free of Maedi Visna. To restart the process of becoming disease-free and accredited as such, every adult animal needed to be tested and all the results had to be negative.

Testing six hundred sheep was a long job, partly because they were scattered around several holdings in the area. By halfway through Monday morning, I had finished the first batch and made a start on the second, which was at the main farm. The system there was very good and the handling facilities were excellent, which made the undertaking very much easier than it often was. There were plenty of assistants on hand to catch and hold each animal, so my job was simply to take blood from the jugular vein of each of my woolly patients and write its ear tag number in a book, alongside the number from the side of the tube containing the blood sample. In this way each sample could be matched to the appropriate sheep.

The handling pen was the same area in which the sheep would have been dipped in years gone by, to prevent sheep scab (a nasty skin disease caused by a mite) and to limit the effects of blowfly strike during the summer. The dipping of sheep is not really practised any more. The strong chemicals that were used have now been banned (unless you hold a specific licence) and it is very difficult to dispose of them correctly. Other, safer methods of control have been developed, but the long and deep troughs, which were previously used to submerge each sheep, still exist at the site of most sheep-handling facilities. Here, the dip was just on the other side of a wooden gate close to where I was working. It had long since fallen into disuse, but had not been drained of the noxious fluid. Layers of dead leaves had fallen onto the surface of the liquid and, partly decomposed, had formed a large and thick mat covering the whole of the dipping area. The recent fall of autumn leaves, made worse by heavy rain, had caused the edges to merge with the surrounding ground and the fetid liquid underneath was perfectly disguised.

It could not have been a more brilliantly conceived trap and it is not difficult to imagine what happened when I leapt over the gate so I could deposit my first polystyrene box of fifty blood-filled glass tubes safely on the passenger seat of my car. I always liked to put a full box of tubes out of the way to avoid the risk of them being knocked over and smashed. I hurdled the gate and both my feet landed on what I thought would be solid ground. Then, everything happened in slow motion. I plunged, without warning, up to my neck in the foul-smelling black soup of sheep dip and rotting leaves, which bore little resemblance to anything I had been submerged in before. I clambered out, soggy and smelly, to peals of laughter from everyone standing nearby.

'Oh yes, I was just about to say,' the farmer called from the other side of the gate.

'Watch out for the sheep dip. You'd never know it was there, hidden under all those leaves — which reminds me, we really must sort that out!'

★ ★ ★

More sheep took up the second part of my week and more testing was required. Wayne, a young farmer who I knew well, had found a couple of dead sheep in one of his fields during the weekend. He had put these deaths down to pneumonia, brought on by the bad weather that had recently affected the area. Heavy rain and strong winds had caused flooding in parts of North Yorkshire. Sheep can easily tolerate cold weather, with their thick woolly fleeces, but they detest rain, in particular persistent, heavy rain, which can permeate their lanolin-coated wool, leaving them cold and miserable. But, when he found another half dozen dead a few days later, Wayne was worried. He usually had a keen attention to detail but he couldn't work out what was going wrong, so he asked me to have a look at the flock.

The affected sheep were from a batch of weaned lambs that had been born in the springtime. They were now about six months old and had grown big and strong, on a combination of their mothers' milk and the summer grass that grew thick and green in the pastures along the side of the River Swale. A farmer who had a holding just three miles downstream from Wayne's farm had once told me that this land was some of the best farming land in the country. The mineral-rich water that came down from the hills at the top of Swaledale, around Muker, Keld, Reeth and other such lovely places, brought vitality to the fields along the length of the river. In the autumn lamb sales at Thirsk Auction Mart, Wayne's sheep would always be amongst the best.

When I arrived, he and his father had already gathered the young sheep into a small paddock adjacent to a holding pen, which would enable me to examine the affected animals and take any samples that I deemed necessary. His lambs did not look as they usually did — some were healthy, but about a third of them were thinner than they should have been and eight out of the group of three hundred had died. The sales were coming up, but it was looking unlikely that any of the lambs would be achieving the top prices to which Wayne was accustomed.

I launched into my usual questioning, probing for clues. In the recent heavy rain, the pastures close to the river had flooded, necessitating a temporary move for the lambs. However, once the floodwaters had subsided, Wayne had moved the flock back to the riverside. I pressed him for more details on the condition of the fields. They were not waterlogged, he reported, and the flood-water had receded several days before the sheep had been moved back onto them. The land had drained well and was not at all boggy. This was a crucial piece of information, because parasitism by liver fluke was at the top of my list of ideas. Sheep can acquire this nasty parasite from grazing on waterlogged fields, especially in autumn, and we had seen a sharp increase in cases in recent years. In fact, until recently we never really saw cases of liver fluke on the eastern side of the Pennines. However, the increasingly wet weather in summer and autumn, attributed to global warming and climate change, has meant that the condition has now become quite common, rather than a rarity.

I examined a few of the thinnest animals, but there wasn't much to see. The next step towards an accurate diagnosis was quite obvious. A post mortem examination was required. I phoned the lab to let them know that Wayne was on his way with three of the recently deceased lambs. We were both anxious to get the answer as soon as possible. We didn't want any more deaths.

Later that afternoon, I received a phone call. It was Gary from the lab again, full of the excitement that I had come to expect from this pathologist when he was on the trail of a diagnosis.

'Hello, Julian!' he said cheerfully. 'It looks like acute pasteurellosis! The lungs are purple with haemorrhage. Have these lambs had any vaccines?'

I confirmed that yes — they had received the correct vaccinations, at the correct time. Wayne was as diligent as any farmer I knew.

'Hmm, well.' This had put a slight damper on Gary's excitement. 'Sometimes disease can break through against a vaccinal titre. It has been awful weather recently. I think I might have developed pneumonia if I'd been out in weather like this! We're running some more tests, just to confirm. I'll keep you posted . . . Oh, another thing — the livers were all clear. Not a trace of fluke, so we're clear on that one!'

I wasn't convinced by the diagnosis of pasteurellosis, although Gary clearly was. He had seen the lungs though, and that was his job, after all. I called Wayne to check the vaccine history again. He confirmed that not only had the vaccines been done, as always, at the correct time, but the sheep had also received an extra dose only three weeks previously, in anticipation of the weather. This 'back end' had been a wet one so far! I advised him to give a precautionary course of antibiotics to any sheep that looked poorly and also to move them onto another pasture. The second part of this advice was risky — moving sheep from place to place can precipitate disease crises through stress. Pasteurellosis — our 'working' diagnosis — could even be triggered by moving sheep from one field to another. Wayne also knew this, but we both agreed it would be sensible, just in case the grazing itself was the cause of the problem.

Three days later, Wayne had done all he had been advised. He had moved the lambs and injected about a hundred sheep with antibiotics in a bid to prevent them from getting any worse, but there had still been more deaths. We had been in contact twice a day by telephone, while we awaited the final test results from the lab. The phone call came halfway through Monday morning, and changed our diagnosis immediately.

'It's lead poisoning! Definitely lead,' explained Gary.

Toxicological testing on the kidneys and liver had revealed dangerously high levels of the heavy metal in the organs of each of the three lambs sent in. The fax confirming this quickly followed the phone call. Despite the relief of having a definitive diagnosis, the gloomy headings on the top of each page did nothing to lighten my mood.

Lamb 1: Lead poisoning with secondary pneumonia.
Lamb 2: Lead poisoning, minimal secondary pneumonia and nephrosis.
Lamb 3: Lead poisoning, mild secondary nephrosis.
Diagnosis: LEAD POISONING.

How had these lambs, grazing the fertile fields alongside the Swale, been exposed to lead? I did some more research before calling Wayne with the news, and what I discovered was more a lesson in geology than in veterinary epidemiology. In years gone by, the landscape of parts of the Dales was not only rural but also industrial. The scattered ruins of lead mines can still be seen in many places. The recent heavy rain had resulted in large quantities of water washing through the lead seams of upper Swaledale, from where the River Swale originated. This water, contaminated by high levels of the toxic mineral, in the form of silt containing lead ore, ran off the hills and into the river. As the river burst its banks further downstream, the silt that had been held in the current was deposited onto the fields where Wayne's sheep had been grazing. The hungry lambs, cropping the grass short and therefore taking in silt as well, had eaten sufficient quantities to damage their internal organs and destroy their blood cells.

Wayne immediately made sure all his lambs were safely inside, away from the dangerous grass. There was no practical cure that could be administered to the lambs. The only drug that might have been helpful needed to be injected intravenously every day, into every sheep, for about five days, which was completely unfeasible given the size of the flock. Wayne and his lambs would just have to sit it out and wait for the lead to leach out of both the lambs and the grass.

The disaster had been contained, although it took many more tests and was quite some time before the lambs were safe for human consumption. The farm next to the River Swale would not be grazing sheep on recently flooded fields again.

★ ★ ★

It did not take long before I was drawing upon my newfound knowledge elsewhere. Only two miles downstream and two weeks later, I found another case of lead poisoning, this time in a herd of Simmental cattle.

The sight in Gordon's fold yard was a sorry one. It was full of about forty year-old store cattle. Gordon had purchased them from nearby hill farms, where they had been overwintered on barley. He fattened these animals on the plentiful grass in the fields around the confluence of Cod Beck with the Swale. The cattle, which were usually a picture of health, with white and deep tan markings, did not look so good. Gordon pointed out about six who were standing, ears down, staring into space and not moving at all. It was otherwise a beautiful autumn afternoon. The sun was doing its best to provide some end-of-season warmth before it slipped out of sight. Gordon explained all, pre-empting my questions. The Simmentals had arrived about three weeks before. The weather was still good and, in the autumn sun, the land nearby his farm had dried out after the recent flooding. The cattle had enjoyed an Indian summer — admittedly one punctuated by an Indian-style monsoon — finishing off the last of the grass. They had obviously tucked into it with some enthusiasm as it would have been vastly superior to anything they had experienced before, coming as they did from upland farms.

'It was just this morning that I didn't think they looked quite right. So I spent an hour or so getting 'em all in, so I could have a closer look.' Gordon was tense. 'It's just those six really. I'd be hard pushed to say that there is much wrong

235

with the others. I thought you'd better come and have a look. You're the vet, you should know what's up wi' 'em. I don't want to lose any — they cost me a fortune. Stores like this are not ten a penny. If I lose any, well, it's my profit gone, you see.'

The more Gordon spoke, the more I felt the pressure rising. I thought I had better interject.

'Where exactly were they grazing, Gordon?'

I hoped that he would point to a field right next to the river.

'Well, everywhere really. All those fields down there.' As we stood on a mound just outside the farmhouse, Gordon pointed out the extent of the grazing which, luckily for me and my diagnosis, included large tracts of land right along the banks of the river. And yes, they too, had been completely flooded about four weeks before.

'The flooding's been bad here,' he explained. 'You see, where Cod Beck joins the Swale, the water sort of backs up and it goes everywhere. Especially if it's been over-wet in the Hambleton Hills as well as the Dales.'

We went back inside to have a closer look at the sick animals. In contrast to lead poisoning in sheep, which usually manifests itself as sudden death, in cattle the disease progresses more slowly. The affected animals develop neurological signs, most frequently characterized by loss of vision. Sure enough, on close examination, these Simmentals were following the textbook perfectly. They were all blind. I confidently pronounced my diagnosis of lead poisoning. It did not impress Gordon as much as I had hoped.

236

The farmer was sceptical.

'Well, we've had this farm for generations and I've never heard of anything like this before. Could it not be pneumonia?'

I explained the signs and my theory, as we examined each blind animal. There was nothing to suggest it might be pneumonia, but there was also no definitive test, other than post mortem examination, to confirm that it was lead poisoning. There were no suitable candidates for post mortem at the moment, and to wait until there was one might be leaving it too late for the possibility of curing the others. Gordon's mood and his confidence in my diagnosis were lifted slightly when I explained that treatment might be feasible for this small number of beasts, if we gave it straight away. We would need to inject a drug called calcium edetate intravenously, every day for about five days. Gordon's demeanour drooped again. Five daily visits from the vet and probably lots of bottles of medicine sounded expensive. I felt somewhat despondent. I had made a pretty good diagnosis (without the need for any expensive lab tests), offered a treatment that would very likely save the lives of all his animals (which he had already pointed out were very valuable and that he couldn't afford to lose) and I had offered to treat them every day until they were cured. I didn't know what more I could do.

I explained it all again and Gordon wandered off into the corner of the fold yard to contemplate the situation. After what seemed like an hour, he stomped back to the cattle crush where I was waiting, and nodded his head.

'You'd better get on with it then. I don't want 'em to die.'

And so I sprung into action, injecting the life-saving medicine into each of the stricken animals. This was what being a vet was all about for me — making a diagnosis and administering a cure. I was in my element. It was so much better than falling into a sheep dip!

Maybe this 'back end' wouldn't be so bad after all!

The Farmer from the West Riding

'There's a man on the phone who wants to speak to you about his goats,' called Zoe, our newly qualified veterinary nurse.

Zoe was chuckling as I hung up my coat. It was before eight thirty and I was the first vet to arrive. A call this early was either because there was a serious problem or it was an anxious farmer.

'He keeps phoning but he's missed you every time and he won't leave a message,' Zoe went on. 'He was on the phone at least three times yesterday. I don't think he is from round here, judging by his accent. I can't really tell what he's talking about, to be honest. Can you speak to him now? I think it would be good if you could. He's very keen to speak to you and he's very persistent.'

It looked as if my first patient of the day would have to wait until I had spoken to the goat farmer, so I took the receiver and introduced myself.

'Argh, nar then. Thank yer fo' coming to spake with me. I'm Rodney. Thing is, like, I need a vet who knows abart goats. And sheep and, well, to tell yer truth, I've seen yer on telly and I thought yer were raight up my street. What I want to ask is — will yer be me vet?'

I was taken aback by this direct approach, especially because I could pinpoint the accent of

239

the goat farmer to within an area of about five miles. He was not from North Yorkshire, but from the West Riding where I grew up, and I could tell he hailed from somewhere slightly to the southwest of Leeds. I asked Rodney the whereabouts of his farm. At Skeldale, we try not to travel long distances to farms, preferring to offer an attentive service to our local farmers. Hours spent on the road make it difficult to guarantee we can attend an emergency promptly. Rodney's farm, as I suspected, was between Leeds and Dewsbury. It was in one of the few remaining patches of rural greenness that hung on as stubbornly as Rodney obviously did, in the face of the urban sprawl.

'It's a bit far out of our normal patch, Rodney,' I explained.

'Aw, go on! We don't have many call outs 'cos me and me son, Matthew, are good at lambing, yer see. I'll bring me sheep and me goats up to you. They'll fit in me car boot no problem.'

I couldn't argue with this. My family lived not far from Rodney's farm, so I knew that the journey to Thirsk would not take more than about fifty minutes. Slightly against my better judgement, I agreed to see Rodney's animals.

'Super,' he said. 'Can I bring me little goats up to see yer? They need their horn buds tekken off. I can come up anytime. Just let me know when. I love me little goats, I do. I've got abart twenty in all and the little uns'll need their horn buds out and . . . '

It was difficult to interrupt a farmer from West Yorkshire when he was on a roll, but the waiting

240

room was filling up with my morning appointments. I needed to bring the conversation to a close more quickly than Rodney did, so I arranged for him to bring his goats up the following week. It was to be the start of a great friendship.

He arrived at the surgery for his appointment, and bundled a riotous gang of about six or seven goat kids out of his car and into my consulting room. Goats are very sensitive to local anaesthetic, so disbudding needs to be performed under full general anaesthetic, by masking the little animals with gas and oxygen. There is a big risk involved, due to unavoidable proximity of the red-hot disbudding iron to the flow of oxygen from the anaesthetic machine. I have heard terrible stories of whole guinea pigs going up in flames when the thermocautery machine has been used too close to the gas supply. I did not want to return any of Rodney's precious little goats with singed heads. It would not get our relationship off to a good start.

Luckily, there were no such incendiary mishaps today, although one little goat called Abi who had been hand-reared (she was Rodney's favourite) was determined to chew through the gas pipes of the anaesthetic machine and cause general havoc. She was cute and she knew it. She tottered over to investigate each patient as they lay on a fleecy blanket, recovering from their ordeal, and would sit on the backs of each of her friends in turn, before skipping off to have a wee in the middle of the consulting room floor. Needless to say, she was the last to volunteer for the procedure!

Whilst I carefully removed each rubbery bud, so the goat kids would not grow horns with which to cause trouble when they were older, Rodney waited in reception, chatting to Sylvia, the receptionist. Sylvia also loved goats and would come in every so often to check how I was getting on. Rodney told her all about his farm, how he did sheepdog trials and how his favourite dog had once gathered all the sheep off a hill, when all the other dogs had failed. When I went out to tell him that everything had gone well — all buds had been removed and no goats had been set on fire — he was still deep in conversation.

'All t'other farmers wo' playing pop with their dogs. None on 'em had got sheep off of moor like, but our Millie, by gum, what a dog, she'd got all on 'em . . . '

I had to interrupt and hand over the bundle of goat kids.

'By gum, that's a proper job! Thank yer very much. I'm much obliged. Thing is, not all vets know abart goats, but I knew you did. I've seen yer on telly like . . . '

He was clearly delighted by our morning's work and, as we shook hands, I knew we would be meeting again.

★   ★   ★

I had not expected our second meeting to be quite so soon. A month had passed, and Millie, Rodney's old and faithful sheepdog about whom we had all heard, had just finished the last of her autumnal work, doing what she did best

— rounding up the sheep on the hill to separate the ewes from their lambs ready for the autumn lamb sales. She had been working hard and it was clear to Rodney that age was catching up with his faithful friend. He had noticed a large and nasty lump growing around one of Millie's teeth, about the size of a large conker. He had rushed her to the local veterinary surgeon, who had given a grave prognosis, saying that the dog had just a few weeks left to live. Rodney was mortified, reluctant to believe that his faithful companion would not see Christmas, let alone next lambing time. His son, Matthew, had urged him to get a second opinion 'from Goat Man.'

We had another phone conversation and the next day, Millie was brought along to the surgery in the car boot that had previously been full of goat kids. She was a happy dog and wagged her tail constantly throughout my examination, resting her head on my knee as I crouched down to examine her on the floor of my consulting room. Farm dogs do not feel comfortable standing on an examination table so I have always found it better to meet them at their level.

There was a firm, boney growth invading the right side of the very front part of Millie's lower jaw extending up and around the canine tooth. Its surface was beginning to ulcerate and I did not need a biopsy to tell me that this was an aggressive tumour. For Millie to have any chance of survival, the mass would have to be removed, along with part of her jaw, to ensure that none was left behind.

I explained to Rodney what we needed to do.

It was testament to the faith he had in me at this early stage of our friendship that he agreed immediately and without question. Most owners pale at the suggestion that part of their pet's jawbone should be removed. It sounds extremely aggressive surgery fraught with complications and post-operative problems. Indeed, it is not something to undertake lightly but, in this case, there really was no other option. We arranged a date for the operation. It meant another long journey up the A1 for Rodney with our patient, but one that he was clearly very happy to make.

As I met Rodney and Millie in the waiting room a few days later, his anxiety was palpable. I promised to phone him as soon as I was done. The operation, while somewhat gruesome, went well. Some of the nurses and the younger vets gathered to watch, grimacing as the oscillating saw cut through the bone around the tumour. When it is necessary to remove a large part of the mandible, the cut ends of the bone are simply left unattached. This is tolerated remarkably well and, amazingly, the function of the mouth is preserved, in a pain-free way. It is always a surprise to the owner that their pet is not horribly disfigured, even immediately after the operation. In Millie's case, though, after I had removed the tumour, the two healthy ends of the bone were still sufficiently close that I could wire them back together, which was even better. Reconstructing the soft tissues of the mouth was the final part of the operation and it was not long before Millie was lifting her head, as she recovered in a warm and comfy kennel.

I called Rodney to tell him that all was well. Needless to say, he was delighted and very relieved. It was not quite plain sailing from this point, as we still needed to make sure that Millie could eat without discomfort. Would she be able to cope with only part of her jaw?

I need not have worried. Only a few short hours after the operation, in the middle of afternoon surgery, Zoe — who was getting to know Rodney and his animals as well as I was — came rushing from the kennels and knocked on my consulting room door.

'Julian. It's amazing! Millie's eating food, from my hand. It doesn't hurt her at all and she's not spilled any!'

I went to have a look. Sure enough, Millie was sitting up, wagging her tail and licking her lips. I went into her kennel and knelt down next to her. As usual, she rested her head on my knee and lifted her eyes, full of trust. She had done well. The cancer that would otherwise have brought her life to a premature end had been removed, and hopefully she would still be around to gather the sheep for next year's lamb sales.

★　★　★

It was as if Rodney now expected miracles, but the third time I treated one of his animals — this time a strong lamb called, appropriately, Lamby — it seemed unlikely that I would be able to live up to his high expectations. The lamb had been born in the springtime but now it was autumn and Lamby — a gimmer lamb (a young female, the ovine equivalent to a heifer) — was nicely grown and sturdy. She was destined to enter the flock and become one of Rodney's best breeding ewes. But Lamby had developed a big problem. A problem as big as half a cucumber. It was a rectal prolapse. This is a condition whereby the rectum pushes out through the anus, a bit like a sock being turned inside out. Lamby's prolapse was various shades of purple and red and I knew it was serious. I had already replaced it once the previous day and, now that it had come out again, the delicate tissues were looking very damaged. A prolapse that doesn't want to stay put is a difficult proposition.

As Rodney lifted Lamby out of his car boot and carried her into my consulting room, I felt an increasing feeling of despair, wondering what exactly I could do next. To replace the prolapse a second time was risky. The membranes were becoming increasingly thin and friable which meant that rupture was a strong possibility. This would be a disaster. As I lifted Lamby off the table and onto the floor so she didn't leap off (she still was full of energy, the contentment at her head-end belying the serious pathology at her rear) this was exactly what happened. The fragile membrane of her exposed rectum tore, leaving a two-inch long hole, through which her small intestines now spilt. It had become a prolapse within a prolapse.

The appearance of small intestines, with all their verminous determination to escape, from the back of a sheep usually leads a veterinary surgeon to reach very quickly for the strong barbiturate solution used for euthanasia. It is characteristically blue, so that it is not mistaken for anything else, and amongst vets is colloquially referred to as 'blue juice'. I looked at Rodney for guidance. Most farmers that I knew would not have entertained the notion of operating on a sheep in this perilous position, but Rodney was not like most farmers.

'If yo' can fix her, then you'd better crack on. I'll wait artside,' were his final words, giving me the green light to try and save his sheep.

What followed was an hour of extremely tense surgery. I had to resect about eight inches of damaged intestine and suture together the separated ends. It was fraught with the risk of infection and wound breakdown and, realistically, the chances of success were close to zero, but I was in the middle of it now and Rodney expected me to do my best. Miraculously, everything went exactly to plan. Lamby woke up from her anaesthetic without complication and Rodney set off back to Dewsbury before lunchtime, with Lamby looking happily out of the rear window of the car boot. I couldn't possibly charge the procedure out at the normal rate, but I still had to charge Rodney for the medication and materials. Even this probably outweighed Lamby's commercial value. Most farmers would have pointed straight towards the 'blue juice' but not the farmer from the West Riding. I admired the love he had for his animals, and I was glad to have the chance to work with him. The farmer from the West Riding was 'raight up my street' too!

247

Elsie the Sow

Chris was passionate about reviving rare breeds of livestock. His first challenge was with a little-known breed of cattle called Whitebred Shorthorns. According to Chris, these cattle were more rare than the giant panda (I thought this might have been because they lived on a diet of white bread — but apparently not!). The breed was a distant relative of the Beef Shorthorn, which ironically was enjoying a surge in popularity, in part because of the beautiful marbled beef it produced. The Whitebred version was few in number, but Chris was doing his bit to keep the breed alive. I had dealt with them on a couple of occasions, pregnancy testing the cows and carrying out their routine TB test, but on none of my visits to his new smallholding had I spotted the pig in a pen, in the corner of the cattle shed. Her name was Elsie.

Elsie was an Oxford Sandy and Black — another rare breed, sadly in decline. She had previously been mated with a Gloucester Old Spot boar and the litter of piglets that were asleep next to her lengthy udder looked as delicious as they were cute. They were, indeed, destined to make the finest sausages in North Yorkshire. But Chris had bigger plans for Elsie. She was soon to be mated with a boar of the same breed. The piglets would be retained within the herd, allowing the breed to increase in number. No more babies would end up as sausages. The problem was that finding a suitable boar of the same breed to mate with Elsie was not easy. Oxford Sandy and Blacks were few and far between. So, Chris decided to use the alternative method of getting a sow pregnant, namely artificial insemination. Whilst Chris had done some work with pigs in this area before, he wanted some professional assistance and my inseminating skills were called into action.

Inseminating a sow is not as difficult as it sounds. My first experience of this process was while I was a veterinary student, working on a large pig unit quite close to my home. The days were long and it was hard work, but I learnt a huge amount about pigs, including how to inseminate a sow. I also learnt quite a lot about power-washing pig sheds.

Throughout my time there, I was closely supervised by the pigman. Pigmen are quite different to other stockmen. They communicate in their own special way, sometimes more at one with their pigs than their fellow humans. The pigman from whom I learnt my pig husbandry skills, spoke in a mixture of words and grunts. Were it not for the jauntily angled flat cap that never left his head, in the dim light of a fattening shed I think he could have been mistaken for one of the stock to which he attended. I have the greatest of admiration for pigmen. My own grandfather was one himself and he truly loved his pigs. It was his influence that first set me on the path towards veterinary medicine. Every time

I see a pig (which is not as often as it used to be), I think of my grandfather and inwardly thank him for steering me towards the career that I now love so much.

So, some twenty-two years later, the skills I learnt from the grunting pigman from Leeds would be put to use. Chris had organized for the delivery of some semen from an Oxford Sandy and Black Boar, along with all the accoutrements that I would need for the procedure. As I unpacked everything when I arrived at his farm, he related how perplexed the postman had been when he had delivered the parcel. There was a large label on the outside of the box proclaiming 'LIVE SEMEN'. As if this didn't make the parcel unusual enough, there were two corkscrew-shaped catheters taped to the outside.

'Elsie is mad on heat,' Chris said, almost beside himself with excitement. 'I've been sitting on her back and she is not budging an inch! Not even making any noises.'

We both knew that this meant that the timing was exactly right for artificial insemination. The two cardinal signs of a sow being in heat are swelling of the vulva and standing still when the pigman sits on her back. At any other time during the pig's oestrus cycle, she will squeal and make a great commotion if a person (or, more usually, a boar) tries to sit on her back and will immediately run away. Elsie was perfectly happy when Chris put his full weight on her rump. In fact they both looked as if they were quite enjoying it. Elsie made small, contented grunting noises and Chris, for his part, sat astride his favourite sow in a similar way to a cowboy trying to tame a bucking bronco. Most pigmen would sit 'side saddle' to test a sow, but Chris tackled all his tasks with a greater enthusiasm than most. He just needed a cowboy hat and a lasso to complete the rather unusual image.

Meanwhile, I was rifling through the box and reading all the instructions. It was straightforward enough. I just needed to remember if a sow's cervix had a left-handed or a right-handed thread.

Elsie stood quite still, happy with Chris on top. I lubricated the foot-long catheter with the corkscrew end and inserted it as gently as I could. As the screw-shaped end reached her cervix, I twisted the catheter in an anticlockwise direction. All was going smoothly. Elsie was content and Chris was comfortable, although Pete, the Gloucester Old Spot boar, watching from the neighbouring pen was confused and disappointed that he was not being called into action today. I held the catheter in place with one hand, and had the bottle of semen in the other. The only way I could remove the sealed cap from the bottle was to snap it off with my teeth. I've done this many times before when I haven't had enough hands, but never with a bottle of pig semen. I had not appreciated that the bottle was slightly pressurized. As I twisted the top off, a squirt of watery semen shot out of the bottle, straight into my face. It then dribbled down onto my waterproof trousers, covering me in precious Oxford Sandy and Black

251

pig semen. There was, thankfully, plenty left in the bottle for Elsie. Chris and his wife, who had also come along to watch the spectacle, could not contain their mirth. I, however, dared not laugh, or even speak, for fear of the stuff trickling into my mouth.

Apart from this minor spillage, most of the contents of the bottle went into the correct place and, after unscrewing the catheter, we sat back and waited for nature to do its thing.

Three months, three weeks and three days later, we had the result that we wanted. Elsie had a litter of beautiful piglets. When they were a week old, I called at the farm to check them over. It was a cold and crisp autumn day, but the piglets were snuggled cosily under a heat lamp beside Elsie. They were a rich ginger colour with black spots, all healthy and strong, destined to perpetuate the breed line and fly the flag for the Oxford Sandy and Black breed. They looked beautifully content and, as I checked each piglet in turn, I felt like a proud father.

Chris was bitten by the breeding bug and had bigger plans afoot. He managed to buy an Oxford Sandy and Black boar from a fellow enthusiast in the south. He phoned to tell me all about it. Donald the boar would be arriving (with his gilt friend Ivana) in a few weeks' time. I was slightly disappointed that I would not be fathering another litter in the same way, but I felt sure that the new Oxford Sandy and Black boar would do just as good a job as me, with my catheter and a plastic bottle from Ireland. I met Donald soon after his arrival and my involvement in the ensuing love triangle continued in a rather peculiar way.

Donald was a handsome but belligerent boar when he first arrived on the farm, throwing his weight around as if issuing the pig equivalent of presidential decrees on a daily basis. Chris's trousers were testament to this, as Donald's sharp and dangerous tusks had made several large holes. Fearing for everyone's safety, Chris arranged for me to call and remove the offending tusks. This is a simple job, although it requires some sedation to keep the patient still whilst the lower tusks are sawn off neatly, using special wire. The procedure is painless, as there are no nerves in the tusks, and the result is a boar who cannot damage the sows when he mates and does not injure the pigman or his trousers.

All went surprisingly smoothly, with much less commotion from Donald than either Chris or I expected. Usually, any job involving injecting a pig includes lots of squealing and charging about, but not so today. Donald trundled off into the corner of his pen to sleep off the rest of his sedative, and I happily drove back to the surgery, ready to regale my colleagues with how successful and straightforward the procedure had been.

So I was not expecting the anxious email that arrived from Chris, two weeks later. Donald had lost his libido. Ever since the tusks had been removed, he had simply laid around, not interested in the seasons of either Ivana or Elsie or any other sow in heat. It was as if the removal of his tusks had emasculated him. At first I thought Chris was joking — his comments about trying soft music and a romantic meal suggested the problem was a minor inconvenience — but the photos that followed showed a pair of shrunken, prune-like testicles and confirmed that the loss of libido was genuine. I was baffled. But, whilst I was as concerned as Chris about this latest turn of events, it did at least mean that maybe I would get another chance to be surrogate father to a litter of Elsie's lovely piglets!

Two Sisters and a Cat

My heart sank when I saw what was in store for me today. It was a home visit to see a geriatric cat called Cedric. It wasn't so much Cedric that was the source of my woe, but his equally geriatric owners, Beryl and Mavis. I had met them a couple of times before. They would come to the practice together, to bring Cedric in for his annual check-ups. However, more recently, the elderly sisters had found it a struggle to get Cedric into a basket and into the car, so their trips to the surgery had become less frequent and, instead, we would visit them at home whenever the cat needed attention. They lived together in the quaint village of Kilburn, at the foot of the escarpment that is dominated by the famous White Horse.

The White Horse is not one of those prehistoric symbols or ancient Celtic sites. It was cut out of the hillside in 1857. It is commonly attributed to the local school teacher John Hodgson and his pupils, although others give the credit to a London businessman and native of Kilburn called Thomas Taylor. Whoever was responsible, it was an impressive feat, as the underlying sandstone is not white at all, and had to be covered with tonnes of limestone chippings to emulate the appearance of those mysterious figures carved out of the chalk downs in other parts of the country. Every so often it is renovated, to keep it white and to stop the limestone subsiding down the hill to its feet. It is always a welcome sight when it comes into view at the end of a long journey, driving up from the south, as it means we are nearly home.

But back to Cedric.

His health was deteriorating and the requirement for home visits had increased sharply over recent months. Today's visit would be a challenge, as usual. Cedric was constipated and it was my job to solve his problem.

There was the smell of wood smoke lingering around the village. It was a beautifully clear autumn day with no wind at all. It was cold, so nearly all the cottages had fires burning in their hearths, and the smoke rose vertically from their chimneys, unhindered by any breeze. I took a deep breath of the sharp, smoky air, and took a moment to survey the amazing browns, reds and oranges of the autumn leaves on the trees that clung to the steep hillside, then I braced myself and strode purposefully up to the cottage and knocked at the door.

'Oh hello, Peter!' shouted Beryl when she finally realized that there was a vet standing on the doorstep. 'Come in. Cedric is in here. He's behind the piano. Mavis can't get him out.'

Cautiously, I entered the little stone cottage to find Mavis sitting on the piano stool with no cat to be seen. The two old sisters had a comical way of bickering between themselves, which always amused me. They also both wore absurdly obvious wigs. Whilst it was not entirely unusual in that era for an old lady to wear a wig, somehow two together in the same small cottage

256

seemed to be just a bit too much wig.

'Peter's come to have a look at Cedric,' explained Beryl to her sister, loudly.

'That's not Peter, is it? Peter's tall,' replied Mavis, at a normal volume.

'Don't be daft. Peter's not small. It is Peter, isn't it?' bellowed Beryl, and she turned to squint back at me to get a better look. 'Oh, you're right,' she continued, at top volume. 'It's not Peter. Mavis, it's not Peter. It's that other one. What's his name?'

'Beryl, that's Julian. He's the other one. He came last time, you remember, when Cedric got the tick on his head. He's the nice one, you must remember? He's been a few times.'

The conversation continued between the sisters, just as if I wasn't there. I thought I should interject, mainly to make my presence felt. At least now I didn't need to confirm who I was.

'Hello, ladies. How is Cedric today?'

I knew he was constipated from the message in the daybook, but I wanted to check, just in case his symptoms had changed in the thirty minutes that had elapsed between their phone call to the surgery and my arrival at their cottage.

Thankfully, it was Mavis who spoke first to explain the problem, as she was the sister who spoke with clarity and at a normal volume.

'He's constipated, you see. He usually goes out to the toilet — out there in that flowerbed, actually.' Mavis pointed out of the window. 'He's such a good cat. I watch him digging his little hole and then scooping soil to cover everything up. It's just as if he has his own little trowel. He's ever so clean. It's quite funny really, when you think about it, isn't it?'

Mavis digressed briefly, then returned to the point. 'But he has started going to his litter tray out there in the porch. He just sits there, pushing and pushing but nothing comes out. Sometimes, he pushes so much I think his eyes are going to pop out.'

Mavis was starting to chuckle now. It was as if explaining the pooing habits of their elderly cat to a much younger, male stranger was quite inappropriate.

'I see. And does he manage to get anything out at all?' I asked.

I knew I needed to glean as much information as I could by asking questions because, at this rate, I did not fancy my chances of getting hold of my patient for an examination. I was anxious to find out if he was straining to pass faeces or urine. It was true that bladder disease could easily be mistaken for constipation, even by very observant owners. Since at least one of the ladies had mistaken *my* identity, I was aware that this was a real possibility. Treating a constipated cat is very different to treating a cat with bladder disease, so it was important that I could differentiate the two.

'Only little bits,' shouted Beryl. 'They look like bits of sheep poo,' she continued, as if she were informing the neighbours at the other end of the village.

'Do stop shouting, Beryl!' pleaded her sister. 'Everyone in the village doesn't want to know about the toilet habits of our cat!'

So, it was clear that Cedric was, indeed, constipated. But to what extent, I could not establish without capturing him. The next challenge was to get him out from his hiding place from either under or behind the piano.

'Right, ladies, I need to examine Cedric. Do you think we will be able to get him out?' I asked with false optimism.

'Mavis. Can you get him out?' shouted Beryl.

It was obviously the job of the younger sister to get down on the floor to persuade the reluctant Cedric out from his hiding place and into the open space of the sitting room carpet.

'Well, I'll try, but he doesn't look keen to come out and say hello,' Mavis said, not sounding very hopeful.

Tempting a shy cat from his hiding place is not an easy thing to do and the tactic of using tasty treats or fancy cat food does not work. I knew that the sisters' plan of lining up various saucers would not tempt Cedric. An old cat is a wise cat and he sensed something was amiss. So the next twenty minutes, which were filled with the opening of lots of packets and tins, were a complete waste of time. Cedric could not be tempted. We needed a plan B.

I peered behind the piano with my head pressed against the musty wall. Using just my left eye, I could make out the vague form of a black and white face, with wide, mottled eyes staring back at me. There was not much space in the hiding place and his feline face was just as contorted as the human one staring, hopefully, down at him.

'I don't think I can reach him, Mavis,' I explained, once I had assessed his position.

He was right in the middle and my arms were not long enough to even touch the tips of his ears. Even if I could have reached, there was no space to grab him and Cedric would surely cling to the carpet or the back of the piano with his claws if I did manage to get him.

The piano was heavy and impossible to move more than just a few inches, so it could not be shifted easily. Maybe I could shuffle it out, just enough to reach him? It was worth a go. But after some grunting and groaning, the gap behind the piano had opened up only enough for me to see Cedric with both my eyes rather than just one. He had shuffled further backwards so he was actually further away from me than he had been before. Clearly I couldn't examine him, and certainly administering an enema from such a distance was not going to happen.

Plan B would not involve grabbing the cat from here. The three humans had a conflab to discuss what form plan B should take. It would either involve using the handle of a mop to poke the cat out, or the stealthy tactic of me leaving, waiting for Cedric to emerge in his own time and then the sisters shutting him in a room without a piano. I didn't want to prod the cat with a mop handle if I could avoid it, and with discretion being the better part of valour, we opted for the latter plan B. Admitting defeat, I skulked out of the cottage and retreated back to the surgery. I had achieved nothing useful so far this morning and I would have to wait for the phone call telling me that Cedric had emerged from his hiding place and had been shut in the kitchen, from where I could lift him onto the kitchen table, check him over and stick an enema up his bottom.

The phone call came about five minutes after I had arrived back at the practice. Cedric was now in the kitchen, so I was soon back on the road, winding my way to Kilburn again. I couldn't help thinking that people would *pay* to travel up and down these beautiful roads on such a glorious autumnal day. I got to call it work. Even if I was unlucky at catching cats, I still considered myself very fortunate.

It was déjà vu, knocking on the cottage door again, although this time Beryl recognized me immediately. I was pleased that I had not been forgotten.

'We've got him in the kitchen,' Beryl bellowed. 'He's behind the fridge!'

'Oh bugger!' were the first words to pass through my mind. At this rate, my whole day would be wasted trying to retrieve this pesky cat from his various hiding places behind pieces of furniture and household appliances. I was not amused. However, as I put my box of equipment on the table, I realized the fridge would be easy to move. It was also one of just a few hiding places. It didn't take long to grab him, and soon Cedric was on the kitchen table.

He was not exactly relaxed or happy to be there, but from here on things were fairly plain sailing. My usual examination of a cat starts at the head end, checking mouth, teeth and gums and looking for any signs that might alert me to underlying disease — pallor of the gums, ulcers in the mouth and so on. Next comes the chest. I listen with a stethoscope to check the heart for rate and rhythm and for murmurs or irregularities, and the lungs for abnormal noises. Then I palpate the abdomen. In a cat, because of its size, it is possible to feel all the different abdominal organs. Today, even the untrained fingers of Mavis or Beryl could easily have identified the problem. Cedric's large intestine was, as I expected, full of rock-hard faeces, with the texture of concrete embedded with small pieces of pebble. He was well and truly constipated, and in need of an enema. I reached into my box of equipment for the little carton that said 'Micralax' on the side. I had never administered an enema on a kitchen table before, but it seemed better than doing it behind the fridge or under the piano.

The name Micralax suggests that the product is small — and it is, if you are a human, for whom it is designed. However, it is not so small if you are a four-kilogram cat. The result of a Micralax enema can be dramatic and highly effective at relieving constipation in any of our small animal patients. I squirted the enema up Cedric's bottom, without any problems. As he jumped off the table, in equal measure disgusted and surprised at what I had just done, I explained to the sisters what would happen next and, in particular, how important it was that Cedric either went straight outside or had constant access to a litter tray. Beryl, who could not hear anything I was saying, promptly opened the sitting room door just as Cedric trotted towards it. My last glimpse of him was of the end of his tail, as he shot back to his favourite hiding place under the piano.

I just hoped the effects of the enema would not be immediate, for the result would be as impossible to remove as its depositor was earlier this morning, and no amount of tasty cat food would tempt it out!

'Hello, Dougie'

Dougie's reputation for being difficult to handle preceded him. As soon as I set eyes on this handsome Amazonian Green Parrot, I knew that trying to do anything with him would pose a somewhat frightening challenge.

I hadn't met Dougie or his doting owner Margaret before. However, I had come across Margaret's ex-husband John several times, with his brilliant little terrier, whose name was Ozzy. John had rescued Ozzy when he was about eight months old. He was a leggy Jack Russell terrier with a rough, wiry coat and was just my kind of dog. Some terriers like to try to show the vet 'who's the boss', and an examination can be a confrontational affair, but there was none of this with Ozzy. He would stand confidently on my consulting room table, wagging his tail, quietly letting me examine him all over and give him his injections without a hint of concern. I congratulated John on giving a home to such a wonderful little dog.

'You've got a grand one there, Mr Hullah,' I commented, although it was clear that any such words were unnecessary. John knew this already.

'Yes, he's a beauty, isn't he?'

Ozzy was a picture of canine health, and rarely needed my veterinary skills, but I looked forward to seeing him once a year for his annual vaccinations. When our patients have significant illnesses or they need regular attention at our clinic, for example after an accident or a big operation, we get to know their owners very well and often become great friends. But although my appointments with Ozzy were infrequent, I felt I had a rapport with John and his dog, as John always made his appointment specifically to see me. Since Ozzy never needed much in the way of veterinary attention, our ten-minute appointment slot was mostly filled with chat. On the occasion of our latest meeting, Ozzy was just as healthy as ever. The only difference I noticed was that John's address had changed. He had moved house to Northallerton, a bustling metropolis compared to the village that was their previous home.

'I see you've moved house, John. What's it like living in a big city?' I joked.

'Well, it's okay. I miss my little village, but we had to move. You see, my wife and I have got divorced,' he explained.

This seemed a strange thing to have done at John's time of life. He was surely in his seventies and it seemed an odd time to end a lifelong partnership. John must have sensed my surprise.

'We didn't fall out or anything and we're still good friends — we meet for coffee and lunch twice a week. It's just that we didn't really want to carry on living in the same house. It's fine. Ozzy and I have moved to Northallerton and Margaret, well, she's got Dougie for company. To tell you the truth, she thinks more about that blooming parrot than she ever did about me!'

My ears pricked up. We were in the middle of

265

filming for series three of *The Yorkshire Vet* and I had come to realize that any animals that strayed away from the norm were a hit with the cameras. A bright green parrot with a doting owner had the makings of a good story.

'Wow! That sounds interesting!' I probed, trying not to be too insensitive to John's marital situation. 'What did Ozzy make of the parrot?'

'Not a lot!' replied John, rolling his eyes. 'The dog and the parrot never got on. That was one of the reasons why we split up.'

It sounded as if the bonds between the humans and their animals in this household were stronger than those between husband and wife. This is not as uncommon as you might imagine — I have heard many stories of a husband being relegated to the sofa so that the dog can sleep on the bed, and in some extreme cases, the dog being so protective of one or other spouse that husband and wife cannot have any physical contact at all.

'And what about Dougie?' I continued. 'Is he okay? If ever he needs anything doing, let me know. I'm not a parrot specialist, but I'd be happy to help.'

I was not sure what I was letting myself in for, but it was all in a good cause.

'Well, it's funny you should say that. His claws and beak are very long and Margaret keeps getting injuries to her shoulders and head when he sits on her. She had him to a vet near where she lives but he got so stressed that he nearly died. The vets had to put him in an oxygen tent for nine hours. She is a bit worried about taking him back!'

That sounded serious. Either the nail clipping had caused Dougie to have a serious panic attack, or the vets were being extremely cautious. Nevertheless, I reaffirmed my offer to help.

Margaret was on the phone the very next day, delighted to have found a vet who was prepared to see her beloved parrot. I just had one final question.

'Margaret, I just have to ask — we are filming at the moment for a television series on Channel 5. Would you have any objection to being on telly?'

And so began another fantastic relationship with a member of the Hullah family.

I made Margaret and Dougie an appointment to come into the surgery the following week. We chose a quiet time so that there would be very few people and no terriers in the waiting room that might be a source of stress for the parrot. John would bring Margaret in his car and leave Ozzy at home. The plan was to give Dougie a general anaesthetic in a calm, quiet and quick way, then clip off his sharp bits and pop him back into his cage, to wake up in familiar surroundings with minimal handling, which would hopefully prevent a repeat of his previous near-death experience.

I knew that Laura, one of the producer-directors of *The Yorkshire Vet*, would be very excited about the prospect of filming a parrot, even though the veterinary part of the procedure would not be particularly technical. She arranged to call and see Dougie and Margaret at their home, to get some preliminary shots and make sure they were happy to be involved. Later that day, I received a text message from Laura, brimming over with excitement.

'Dougie is AMAZING! Margaret is lovely and everything in her kitchen is bright green, to match the parrot. And DOUGIE SPEAKS WITH A YORKSHIRE ACCENT!'

A week later, Margaret and John brought Dougie to the surgery, ready for his pedicure and beak trimming. He was in a bright green basket, and Margaret was wearing a bright green coat and colourful parrot earrings. I ushered them into the consulting room, and right on cue, as if following a script, the fantastic green bird looked at me, then looked straight into Laura's camera and shouted, in the broadest of Yorkshire accents, 'Hellorr, Dougie!'

Not for the first time, Laura's camera started wobbling uncontrollably as we all fell about laughing.

When you are a veterinary surgeon, you never have a conversation with your patient — well, not one that involves them actually talking to you in words, anyway. I wasn't quite sure what to do next. It seemed rude not to reply, so I introduced myself.

'Hello, Dougie, I'm Julian.'

'What's up wi' you then?' he responded!

Dougie's chatter continued constantly as Kate, one of our very experienced nurses, manoeuvred him carefully into a smaller basket which we then enveloped in a large plastic bag, to make it into an oxygen tent. In this way we could pipe anaesthetic gas into the cage, so he could gently go to sleep with the minimum of stress. Although we couldn't see him inside the bag, Kate and I both knew when he was asleep. Once the talking stopped, he was ready.

Claws clipped and beak trimmed, Dougie was soon awake, safely in his cage, sitting on his perch and chatting with anyone he met in the waiting room. Margaret was delighted, as was I. The procedure had been uneventful and I had escaped without injury from that powerful beak and those fearsome talons.

Dougie, for his part, became a TV sensation. The most famous parrot in the county. The parrot with a Yorkshire accent!

The Calf that was Automatically Scraped

Autumn was drawing to a close and Simon had just brought his cows in. As soon as the nights cool down, the grass stops growing and the days shorten, dairy cows need to come inside. If the weather stays reasonable, they just come in at night for a few weeks, but by the end of October, they are in all the time. The pastures need to rest and recover, and dairy cows, with their thin skin and sensitive dispositions, need to be protected from the impending change in the weather.

Simon's herd was impeccably organized and the health and welfare of the cows was paramount. These days, some dairy farmers keep their cows inside all year round in an effort to maximize their milk yield, at a time when milk prices are so ridiculously low that it is otherwise almost impossible to make ends meet. Not so on this farm. Each cow had her own name, sometimes inherited from her mother, like 'Daisy the Third' or 'Buttercup the Second' or sometimes unique, like 'Sally' or 'Justine'. This was the way that Simon recorded the identities of his animals when I undertook his fortnightly fertility visits. It made a nice change from a list of numbers. These visits were to ensure that his cows were pregnant and that they went on to calve and restart another ten-month lactation, with as little

270

loss of time as possible. To this end, every cow was scanned for pregnancy, five weeks after she had been inseminated.

The traditional method of pregnancy diagnosis in cattle was to palpate the uterus, per rectum, to feel for a calf (the typical 'hand up a cow's backside' image of the large animal vet), but only the most experienced vets could diagnose a pregnancy reliably as early as thirty-five days. The use of ultrasound scanning has removed the element of doubt, although unfortunately for the vet and the cow, the scanning probe still has to go in by the same route. The uterus can be seen, in black and white and various shades of grey, as can the presence of a calf, floating about in its little sac of amniotic fluid.

During my visit, I would also check cows that had recently calved and scan their ovaries for signs of activity or inactivity. This would tell us if and when they were likely to come back into heat (the term for this in cows is 'bulling'). Once a cow came bulling, it was ready to get back into calf. A cow's ovaries range from the size of a pea to the size of a ping-pong ball. Some are as big as a ping-pong ball but with structures on their surface the size of a pea. The standard size is about that of a broad bean. Every cow has two. Part of the routine examination of a cow for fertility involves finding and feeling each one. I remember, as a student, the daunting prospect of having to find and palpate each ovary, in the never-endingly cavernous insides of a bovine, repeatedly and accurately, cow after cow. It seemed an impossible task, but it is one that a

271

large animal vet needs to be able to do with ease.

There would usually be twenty-five to thirty cows to see when I came, every second Thursday morning. At least, that was what Simon would have told the receptionist when he phoned the surgery, and what it would say in the daybook: 'About twenty. Maybe twenty-five or thirty tops.'

I knew, though, from years of experience that the number he had specified bore very little resemblance to the actual number of cows that I would be examining. I usually packed an extra box of plastic arm-length gloves and another bottle of lubricant, because Simon would always have found some extras by the time I got there.

So as I drove down the bumpy track towards the farm on this foggy autumn morning, I was expecting a raft of 'while you're here' jobs to do either before or after I started the action with my scanner. At this time of year there was usually a bunch of little calves with pneumonia to deal with. The damp fog that descends on the Vale of York in October provides perfect conditions for pneumonic bacteria and viruses to linger, and young calves, taken away from their mothers and put into groups with others of a similar age, are always at risk, in the same way that children in a nursery are constantly sharing a cold.

I pulled up in my usual parking place outside the dairy, climbed into my wellies and put on an extra layer, to protect me from the pervading damp chill of the fog. I was welcomed by Simon stomping towards me, looking agitated.

'Ah, about time. I could have done with you abart an hour ago.'

I checked my watch, although I could tell from the chill and from the fact that the fog had not lifted even slightly that it could not be late. It was exactly half past nine — the time arranged for my visit. I was taken aback. Admittedly, there had been many times when I had been late, delayed by an emergency cat with diarrhoea or a vomiting dog that had arrived without an appointment just as I was about to leave, or indeed a visit to see another batch of pneumonic calves, but today I was bang on time.

'Sorry, Simon. Is there a problem?' I tried to calm him down.

'Well, not now there isn't. But you'll have to have a look at this poor little bloody calf before we start with the cows. I haven't even got 'em sorted yet. What a bloody morning!'

He marched off in the direction of the calf pens. I grabbed some kit and trotted after him, trying to get some more information as we crossed the yard.

'This', he declared, 'is a very lucky calf. A bloody, bloody lucky calf'.

That didn't give me a lot to go on. I was hoping for something a bit more specific — poorly, lame, weak, not eating . . . being lucky didn't help me much. However, as we reached the calf's pen, Simon stood with his hands on his hips and explained, 'Well, this is what happened.'

What Simon described, with some pride, was the amazing story of a heroic rescue. I listened in astonishment, open-mouthed at times.

'This calf should not have been born this morning. It was not due until next week, so I'd put its mum in the cubicle house with all the milking cows, just so she could get used to it. She's a heifer, you see, so I thought it'd be good to let her get used to the cubicles and what not.'

This was good practice and a good idea. First-time calving heifers had no experience of the cubicle housing shed, where the milking cows lived, so introducing them a week or so before their calving date meant they could meet the other cows and become acquainted with the ways of the milking herd gradually, before they calved and before they went into the parlour for the first time.

'I came in this morning, at t'usual time, and I noticed this cow was bawling and she had some cleansing out of her back end,' Simon explained.

This suggested that she had calved, unexpectedly, during the night.

'I looked around for a calf, 'cos I thought it was a bit odd. But there was no calf *anywhere* to be seen. I just could not understand it. It looked just as if she had calved while she were in the cubicles but if she had, she must have been over a week early and, well, I couldn't see a calf anywhere. I looked and looked, but no calf. Then, eventually, I noticed another cow who was bawling even more, at the top end o' the cubicle house, right by the end where the slurry lagoon is. I looked at the automatic scrapers and I just thought, 'Shit — this calf's been automatically scraped into the slurry lagoon,' and so I rushed, at high speed, up to the top of the cubicle house. And I opened the doors and peered into the slurry pit.'

Automatic scrapers are a bit like windscreen wipers for the floor of a cow shed. The cows stand or lie in rows of cubicles, with passageways in between. The cubicles are designed so that when the cow passes faeces, it goes into the passage rather than onto the bedding in the cubicle, and it can then be scraped away. The automatic scraper is attached to a rail or a cable that runs along the passage and it is constantly moving back and forth, sweeping the copious semi-solid by-products of a ruminant's digestion off the floor and into a large lagoon of slurry at the end of the building, often twenty or thirty feet deep. The system is very effective at keeping the standing areas clean because the scraper goes up and down every five or ten minutes, in contrast to the twice-daily scrape that happens if the job is done by the farmer on a little tractor with a scraper on the back. The cows learn very quickly to step over the slowly moving scraper, but a newborn calf would have no idea.

'And when I opened the doors,' exclaimed Simon, clearly reliving the moment, 'I looked down and there was this little calf, bobbing around and *trying to swim* in the shit. All I could see was its poor little nose and I thought, 'Bloody hell, I need to get that little calf out o' there 'cos it'll drown.' That's when I realized I needed a ladder, so I rushed off to get one.'

Simon was animated, although trying to remain as matter-of-fact as he could, under the dramatic circumstances.

'I got a ladder and I put it into the slurry lagoon until it stopped going down,' he explained. I had visions of the ladder simply sliding, effortlessly and endlessly into the thick brown pond, but apparently the slurry lagoon had a concrete bottom. Simon had helped to build it so he knew exactly how deep it was and how long his ladder needed to be.

'Once it was in, I climbed down, with a rope around my neck. I hadn't got time to get our lad or our old man to help, so if I'd have gone in too I think we'd have both been gonners. Anyway it didn't come to that, 'cos I grabbed the calf by its nose — which was the only bit sticking out of the shit — and wrapped my rope round its neck. It was slippery as hell, because it was covered in shit, like, but I managed to get a grip with my rope and I pulled it up and out . . . and this is it.'

Simon waved at a black and white-with-a-hint-of-brown Friesian heifer, which was standing in a pen with a thick dry straw bed, utterly unperturbed by her life-threatening ordeal a mere hour earlier. I checked her over and she seemed remarkably fit, all things considered.

'I've decided to call her 'Bob' even though she's a heifer,' remarked Simon, with a wry smile, which gave way to a massive grin. ''Cos she was bobbing around like a little cork!'

I gave Bob some medication as a precaution against the range of potentially serious illness that she might now face having been submerged in slurry for several hours, but she had indeed been a very, very lucky calf. I hoped I would be meeting her in the future during one of my routine visits. I would chuckle when Simon's list of cows for pregnancy testing had big ticks next to 'Justine', 'Sarah' and 'Bob'. But for now there were still twenty cows to check, or twenty-five, thirty tops.

'Right, now for these cows. Can yer give us a hand?' called Simon. 'I've not sorted any out yet. There's quite a few to do. Forty, maybe fifty. We'd better get cracking.'

Acknowledgements

Writing *Through the Seasons*, as it has come to be known to me and everyone involved in its production, has been every bit as much fun as the writing of my first book, *Horses, Heifers and Hairy Pigs*. Pulling stories out of the back parts of my memory, fitting them together and putting them down on paper, has been another brilliant experience, very much akin to finding an old photo album and perusing its pages. I am grateful to David Riding, from MBA Literary Agents, and Louise Dixon from Michael O'Mara Books for persuading me that this venture was a good idea and that I was capable of writing such a book. You were obviously both right. Again. Thank you!

As before, thank you to my colleagues, clients and their animals for providing me with the subject matter for this book. Without the exuberant and diverse range of clients I have worked with over my career and their quirky pets and farm animals, this book would never have been possible. As we have seen in other, more impressive books in the past, Thirsk has a plentiful supply of characters, human and animal, which have lent themselves to featuring in animal-based stories. It has been the most amazing place to practice veterinary medicine and I have been truly privileged to have had the good fortune to have worked in this amazing little market town for most of my veterinary career. The White Rose Book Cafe sits proudly in the market square, in the middle of Thirsk, and the shop has provided stalwart support for my first book and, judging by the passion and enthusiasm of its owner, Sue Lake, I imagine and hope that the same support will come for *Through the Seasons*. Thank you for the help you have given already and thank you in advance for supporting this book. You have been amazing!

I must thank Maurice Duffield, an archetypal Yorkshire farmer and cricket fanatic, for letting me have photos taken on his lovely farm for the front cover of the book. Moreover to my eldest son, Jack, for taking the jacket pictures! At just fourteen years old, he must be one of the youngest 'professional' photographers to take a front cover shot. On a sunny Sunday in April, we jumped at the chance to get some shots with the correct backdrop; Laura Blair, sorry you missed out — you can *definitely* do the cover for my next book!

The book has been a complete family affair: as well as Jack taking the photos, my sister proofread — thank you for picking up so many typos! My mum and dad have continued to provide moral support but, specifically, thanks to my wife, Anne, for so skilfully and fastidiously editing my words. It seemed to take longer this time: I don't know whether that's because my first drafts were not so good, or because you became more pedantic, but I do know it is now much better than the version that I first knocked out. And thank you to Archie, my youngest son, for being an inspiration to me every day.

We do hope that you have enjoyed reading
this large print book.

Did you know that all of our titles
are available for purchase?

We publish a wide range of high quality
large print books including:
Romances, Mysteries, Classics
General Fiction
Non Fiction and Westerns

Special interest titles available in
large print are:
The Little Oxford Dictionary
Music Book
Song Book
Hymn Book
Service Book

Also available from us courtesy of
Oxford University Press:
Young Readers' Dictionary
(large print edition)
Young Readers' Thesaurus
(large print edition)

For further information or a free
brochure, please contact us at:
Ulverscroft Large Print Books Ltd.,
The Green, Bradgate Road, Anstey,
Leicester, LE7 7FU, England.
Tel: (00 44) 0116 236 4325
Fax: (00 44) 0116 234 0205

Other titles published by Ulverscroft:

HORSES, HEIFERS AND HAIRY PIGS

Julian Norton

The star of a television programme about his life as a Yorkshire vet, Julian Norton works at the relocated practice in Thirsk made famous by James Herriot in his *All Creatures Great and Small* books. From his childhood love of animals, through his training and first steps in the profession and the pressures and challenges faced by vets (such as BSE in the 1990s and foot-and-mouth in 2001), and dealing with unexpected exotic pets — and excitable humans too — Julian has seen all sides of the veterinary world. Just as happy calving a cow, treating a dehydrated kitten or tending to a horse trapped in barbed wire, Julian's tales bring to life the world of the working vet and the highs and lows he and his colleagues face on a daily basis.

READING WITH PATRICK

Michelle Kuo

As a young English teacher keen to make a difference in the world, Michelle Kuo took a job at a tough school in the Mississippi Delta, sharing books and poetry with a young African-American teenager named Patrick and his classmates. For the first time, these kids began to engage with ideas and dreams beyond their small town, and to gain an insight into themselves that they had never had before. Two years later, Michelle left to go to law school; but Patrick began to lose his way, ending up jailed for murder. And that's when Michelle decided that her work was not done, and began to visit Patrick once a week, and soon every day, to read with him again . . .

THE DAY THAT WENT MISSING

Richard Beard

On a family summer holiday in Cornwall in 1978, Nicholas and his brother Richard are jumping in the waves. Suddenly, Nicholas is out of his depth, and drowns. Richard and his older brothers don't attend the funeral; incredibly, the family return immediately to the same cottage to complete the holiday. They soon stop speaking of the catastrophe, and Nicky is written out of the family memory. Nearly forty years later, Richard Beard is haunted by the missing grief of his childhood, but doesn't know the date of the accident or the name of the beach. So he sets out on a painstaking investigation to rebuild Nicky's life, and ultimately to recreate the precise events on the day of the accident. Who was Nicky? Why did the family react as they did? And what actually happened?

ARTHUR

Mikael Lindnord

When you are racing 435 miles through the jungles and mountains of South America, the last thing you need is a stray dog tagging along. But that's exactly what happened to Mikael Lindnord, captain of a Swedish adventure racing team, when he threw a scruffy but dignified mongrel a meatball one afternoon. When they left, the dog followed. Try as they might, they couldn't lose him — and soon Mikael realised he didn't want to. Crossing rivers, battling illness and injury, and struggling through some of the toughest terrain on the planet, the team and the dog walked together towards the finish line, where Mikael decided he would save Arthur and bring him back to his family in Sweden, whatever it took.

SWELL

Jenny Landreth

These days, swimming may seem like the most egalitarian of pastimes, but this wasn't always the case. Even into the twentieth century, women could be arrested and fined if they dared to dive into a lake. It wasn't until the 1930s that they were finally, and reluctantly, granted equal access. But this didn't happen by accident or benevolence, and *Swell* is the story of the women who forced the doors open. It's the story of how swimming can be a barometer for women's equality; a thank-you to the fearless 'swimming suffragettes' who took on the status quo — and won. It's a story of famous women, stars and Olympians, and it's about ordinary women's relationship with water too. It's also the story of how Jenny Landreth eventually came to be a keen swimmer herself.

TARA

Rosemary and Robert Forrester

Robert arrives in Colombia with a surprise for his wife, Rosemary: Tara, a Jack Russell puppy. Join this adventurous couple — and their amazing, seafaring canine crew of one — as they cruise around the world on their yacht, *Deusa*. Their exciting and sometimes hair-raising adventures on land and sea include tales of tsunamis, modern-day pirates, corrupt customs officials, several instances of *'Dog Overboard!'*, many new friends — and near disaster off the Australian coast . . .